Pilates
on
the
Ball

Pilates
on
the
Ball

The World's Most Popular
Workout Using
the Exercise Ball

Colleen Craig

Healing Arts Press
Rochester, Vermont

Healing Arts Press
One Park Street
Rochester, Vermont 05767
www.InnerTraditions.com

Healing Arts Press is a division of Inner Traditions International

Note to the reader: This book is intended as an informational guide. The remedies, approaches, and techniques described herein are meant to supplement, and not to be a substitute for, professional medical care or treatment. They should not be used to treat a serious ailment without prior consultation with a qualified health care professional.

Library of Congress Cataloging-in-Publication Data
Craig, Colleen. 1956–
    Pilates on the ball : the world's most popular workout using the excerise ball / Colleen Craig.
        p. cm.
    ISBN 0-89281-981-2 (book)
    ISBN 0-89281-095-5 (book and DVD)
    1. Pilates method. 2. Medicine ball. I. Title.

RA781 .C666 2001
613.7'1—dc21

                                                    2001039571

Printed and bound in the United States by Capital City Press

10   9   8   7   6   5   4   3   2

Text design by Cindy Sutherland, layout by Cindy Sutherland and Priscilla Baker
This book was typeset in Goudy with Avant Garde as the display typeface

Contents

Preface

The first time I attended a ball class—working out with a large vinyl, air-filled ball—it was at my local Y. I began the class full of energy and self-assurance. After all, you don't fight gravity lying horizontally on a mat. I dazzled myself with rolling and balancing, stretching and lunging, tossing the ball high into the air and catching it between my feet like a circus performer. Wow!

Halfway through the forty-minute class I was out of breath and out of steam. My eyes flitted from the clock to the instructor's face: why was she torturing us? I surveyed the other participants. A couple of them were whining or smiling ironically at their own failings as they surrendered, exhausted, falling to the floor near their balls.

It was rare for me as a partaker in a mind/body class to be concerned with the other participants' progress, but I had to assess how others were coping. Nothing in my physical past, not all the years of dance training, childhood gymnastics competitions, or extensive Pilates training, had quite prepared me for the astonishing vigors of ballwork. Every muscle in my body was alive: even my abdominals, which I believed to be rock hard, were groaning. After the forty-minute class I had planned to go to the weight room but could hardly drag a comb through my hair. Instead I collapsed into a chair in the Y's cafeteria and tried to understand what had happened.

I often boasted of being stronger in my mid-forties than I was in my midtwenties. I claimed that Pilates had realigned and reshaped my body, heightened my mind/body awareness, and cultivated a deep core strength I never believed I possessed. Yet the ball had played havoc with the image I held of myself. During some exercises I had no idea what muscles to recruit in order to accomplish the balance and control needed. For the first time I understood the full significance of the word *recruit*—a word appropriated from military parlance—to describe the physical mobilization of muscles. This word had never meant anything to me in the context of movement classes, but now translated nicely to the challenge of ballwork.

At the same time that I was critically analyzing the ball, I was also savoring the bliss of the workout. Never before had I experienced such deep, comfortable stretches. I had lain backward over the ball and felt my spine become one with the shape of the sphere as the pull of gravity deliciously opened me up bone by bone. Never had I felt such an efficient, functional use of my body. I performed a series of arm exercises in which the entire torso was engaged, not only the arms and shoulders. And near the end of the workout, when we were allowed to drape our spent bodies over our balls and sink into a luscious pose that the instructor dubbed "a little piece of heaven," I had a flash of womblike serenity, with breath as my only companion.

Soon after that fateful first experience I began to take serious stock of the group mat classes that I instructed each week based on the teachings of Joseph Pilates. In a traditional private Pilates session you usually work half the time on the mat and half on an apparatus. Joseph Pilates had designed specific pieces of equipment to add resistance to the matwork and to enhance stretching, both of which are key to an effective bone and muscle workout. Yet these pieces of equipment, found in exclusive Pilates studios around the world, are expensive and not at all portable. In a group situation you are restricted to the mat exercises. This has always seemed like a shortcoming to me. If only I could somehow integrate the ball into my group classes so that the user would get all the benefits of resistance and weight-bearing support right from the start. Moreover, the ball would expose mat students to the repertoire of equipment-based routines.

Exercise balls were not used in my Pilates training and are not part of the equipment associated with the Pilates Method. Yet I had the potential to create something new and to make all that was good about Pilates even more effective for my students. One by one I methodically went through all the mat and equipment-based exercises to determine which exercises the ball could enhance. Unlike the Y class with its grueling repetitions and aerobic emphasis, I tried to stay as close as possible to my extensive Pilates training and experience, remaining as faithful as I could to the science and principles of the method. When I began to share Pilates on the Ball with other Pilates teachers, physiotherapists, physical education teachers, and fitness editors, their overwhelming response confirmed what I already knew—that I was on to something good.

However, it was only when I began to teach Pilates on the Ball to many different students, all of different ages and fitness levels, that I fully appreciated how miraculous the exercise ball is. Even nonathletic, sedentary adults gleefully crawled on their hands and knees and performed a series of lusty push-ups. The demands of the ball and how it taught them to move with the whole body amazed elite athletes. People could connect to the ball in ways that were not possible with a machine or a mat and were discovering in this movement method exactly what they wanted from exercise.

Working with the ball was fun yet transforming, vigorous yet safe—a method that addressed the spine, waistline, muscle tone, flexibility, *and* ability to relax. What was it that spoke so totally to the whole body? And the big, beautiful air-filled balls! Just the look of them made adults' faces light up with anticipation.

In the end, the experience of pleasure may be the most significant aspect that the ball brings to any session. Notwithstanding the highly impressive deep-body conditioning, the cardiovascular and postural benefits, and the remarkable balance and coordination practice, the ball is really not so much about exercise as it is about play. The ball breaks up our adult habits and judgments, soothes our physical and emotional wounds, and reconnects us with childhood, or at least to a part of us that is younger, freer, and unburdened.

The ball plays shamelessly with gravity to create a double kick of pleasure and danger. I wonder sometimes as I slowly roll over the curve of my ball, head over tail, or backward into a deep expansion that opens my heart to the sky, if this is not how it must feel to tumble weightlessly in space.

Introduction

Heaven or Hell?
Our Relationship to Physical Activity

*Whenever I feel
like exercise, I lie down
until the feeling passes.*
—Robert Maynard
Hutchins

Ingrid's Story

On a recent trip to Africa I had tea with Ingrid, a seventy-year-old widow of
a European diplomat. My friends and I sat outside on a veranda overlooking a
sprawling garden wild with climbers, fig trees, and unswept leaves, an oasis
where even in the dead of an African winter insects, birds, and flowers
thrived. The sun was very sharp but falling fast as the tea arrived, colonial
style, carried on a well-dressed tray by the domestic helper. My friends baited
Ingrid to talk about her sojourns in the various African countries where she
and her late husband had lived. "Sudan, Egypt, Congo, Kenya, Uganda," she
rattled off. She was my mother's age yet had lived a life I could not imagine.
Not a life of shopping malls, PTA meetings, or painting classes, but one of ter-
rorist bombings, grenade attacks, luxury houses on stilts overlooking foreign
oceans; a decadent life with too much drinking and cigarette smoking.

The sharp cold made us move inside. We sat on leather sofas in front of a
massive stone fireplace surrounded by animal-skin carpets and bead-decorated
stools. Every eye was on the sun-aged, blue-eyed diplomat's wife, who smoothed
a stray piece of hair back from her face in a mood reminiscent of a 1950s Hol-
lywood starlet. Once in Uganda she had been roused from a bath at midnight
by the sound of guerillas with AK-47s stomping around in the very next room.
After Idi Amin's fall, Ingrid slipped into the dictator's ransacked home to help
herself to a stool and a telephone. These stories would have had a historian or
a journalist jumping. Yet what made my ears perk up was her announcement

did you know?

- Pilates can improve your posture. You will feel taller.
- Pilates builds long, lean muscles without bulk.
- Pilates improves stamina, coordination, flexibility, and joint mobility.
- Pilates firms abdominals and prevents and heals lower back pain.
- Pilates relaxes and rejuvenates.

of how she had transformed the mammoth stone-filled field around her new home into a lush garden. Her husband, she explained, had died two years previously; soon after she had begun to "shrivel up," and she needed to walk with a cane. One day she looked into a mirror, a crystal glass full of scotch nearby, to admit that she had again gone off the wagon and was old—a "skeleton" living in another radically transformed African country. Then a close friend had helped her to stop drinking. Sober and alone, she was forced to take control of her life.

"What did you do?" I asked.

The fire glowed in the grate behind her. "Physical work—like a man," she said with a small smile. "I designed the garden. I ordered truckloads of dirt. I put in the two fishponds. Of course I had help. I had to get rid of the 'sticks.' These, what-you-call, canes, held me back from planting."

"Now what do you do?" I asked. She had two gardeners who appeared to take care of much of the yard work.

"Swim aerobics," she said. "I started eight months ago. I go every second day. The swim aerobics led to the mall walking."

"Mall walking?"

"On the days I don't swim, I walk. It's very organized. True as God, they even time us with stopwatches. Like an American, I am," she laughed. "Can you see me walking in circles inside a mall? But I love it."

"You do?" exclaimed one of my friends. Like me he was no doubt trying to imagine Ingrid clad in sneakers and track clothing.

Ingrid nodded.

Behind the chair in which she sat Ingrid had arranged some fat purple-brown pods with other dried flowers. I knew these pods opened with a crack—a crack you could hear from a distance—before flinging out their seeds. One look at these wondrous pods and I was reminded of the transforming power of a new beginning.

"My life is saved," Ingrid added after a moment. "My face is old. I am ashamed of my face. But my body, it sings."

Movement and You

What is your relationship to physical activity? Have you despised exercise most of your life so that even the idea of a walk feels like a chore? Or do you crazily toss yourself from one activity to the next, from one new fitness phase to another? Perhaps you are one of the so-called weekend warriors, the people who do nothing physical all week, then at the first opportunity toss themselves into frenzied, extended exercise—pedaling all day on an ill-tuned bicycle or swimming nonstop across a lake. Or maybe you are relatively fit. You are disciplined enough to slip in three sessions a week at your local Y or health club, but you are terribly bored of the same old routine. In frustration you find yourself on the floor, your feet hooked under a heavy bar, forcing yourself to do dozens and dozens of sit-ups. Yet in spite of your efforts you do not achieve the results you want.

Throughout my life I have had the opportunity to live on different continents and learn from different peoples and cultures. In many countries I have witnessed the same erratic relationship to exercise that we North Americans have. In Russia I have seen people worn to the bone by the strains of daily life, as dog-tired as the stray mutts who sleep outside the metro stations; yet these same people will fire off a set of push-ups in their cramped apartments. They may not exercise again for months, even years. In South Africa I have seen activists pull on torn sneakers to jog ten kilometers and then smoke their lungs out at meetings afterward. In North America we use our cars to drive two blocks to a corner store, then we sit atop stationary bikes, often in front of the television, unaware of our posture or technique. In spite of an extensive background in dance movement and ballet, even I cut myself off from my body for twenty years, believing that intellectual pursuits were "noble" and physical ones "superficial."

It is not only our attitudes that make it difficult to sustain a healthy kinship to physical activity. Some of us have physical limitations or are recovering from chronic pain and injuries. We believe that because of a weak knee or ankle we will never be able to bend down to weed the garden or squat for as long as necessary before a child, never mind lie comfortably on our bellies under the tree canopy or roll on to our hands and knees to admire the beauty of our gardens. We are daunted by the thought of trying a new sport because of the fear of aggravating an injury or pulling an unused muscle.

Every day we read a new article or see a television show about the benefits of exercise. We know how splendid we feel after a long walk. We see how fit and graceful are our animals as they luxuriate in their stretches. We know of the studies that attest to the facts that exercise rejuvenates aging bodies, calms stress and anxiety, lowers blood pressure, and lessens the risks of many diseases. Some exercise methods, including Pilates on the Ball, claim to do even more. But the success of any exercise approach relies on the responsibility of the participant, the doer, and how he or she connects to that method mentally, emotionally, and physically. It is my hope that you, like so many others, will fully embrace Pilates on the Ball and let it be an answer to your movement desires.

questions to ponder: what's missing from your workout?

How have you made your exercise choices in the past? We are so influenced by media, friends, and spouses that we sample fitness trends without a sense of what we need.

What is missing from your workout? Intensity? Pleasure? Satisfaction? Challenge? Variety? Relaxation?

What is your reason for exercising? Peer or media pressure? Preventive medicine? Physical therapy to recover lost strength or coordination from a disease or injury?

Do you ever wish, in hindsight, that you could have taken up a particular sport or tried a physical activity? Which ones and why?

What would you ultimately wish to achieve from Pilates on the Ball?

questions to ponder: medical and physical restrictions

What physical restrictions do you have? What injuries or diseases?

Where in the body do you tend to hold stress or experience pain and discomfort?

Have you checked with your doctor or health practitioner to see if you suffer from any health problems or conditions that may stop you from participating in this exercise program?

Who Can Benefit?

This book presents a wide and diverse range of movement possibilities to help you rediscover how to move, stretch, dance, and play healthfully and joyfully. Depending on your fitness level and curiosity, you can learn anything from small healing exercises to very challenging ones. Pilates on the Ball stimulates more than muscles, and many different types of people will benefit. The beginner, staying within modifications and working at his or her own speed, will find ballwork more manageable than many exercise methods. Even the nonexerciser, possibly overweight and previously sedentary, can start by doing a few safe abdominal exercises on the mat and then using the ball to sit on, bounce on, or stretch over. People recovering from injuries and physical restrictions can follow the therapeutic modifications and add more rigorous variations as their strength improves.

Men and women love the intensity and challenge of the ball and will use it as a way to take the tedium out of workouts. More important, the ball breaks existing movement patterns and will help you tap in to an unused pool of muscles to work the "weak" and not just the "strong" side of your body. Like many others, you will probably connect to the ball much more easily than to a machine. The ball adds a gentle resistance to each exercise, which builds long lean muscles, frees up holding patterns, and acts as an excellent stress releaser. Bouncing on the ball is a fun and safe way to lose weight and improve cardiovascular fitness. Dancers and athletes will use Pilates on the Ball to correct alignment problems and balance a body that has relied chronically on certain muscles to perform at the expense of others.

Whether you are a beginner or a professional movement expert, you are ready for the challenge and fun of Pilates on the Ball. Perhaps you are familiar with the Pilates Method but are new to the ball—or familiar with the ball but new to Pilates. Maybe you know nothing about either. You simply want an effective, yet safe, intelligent workout.

Movement with Meaning: The Intelligent Workout

In caveman days our survival depended on physical exertion; today our survival depends on balance, both outside the body and within. When the diplomat's wife, Ingrid, discovered the joy and benefits of movement her life metamorphosed because she added physical activity and cardio endurance to a life previously void of such activities. Many of my students come to my classes seeking physical conditioning, but what they also receive is mental conditioning—a way to get in touch with their inner strength and inner calm and to balance the chaos of their lives with sanity.

Joseph Pilates fused the best aspects of Eastern and Western exercise disciplines, and it is the balancing of both these worlds that binds so many people to his method and makes it the perfect antidote to modern living. From the East he borrowed the philosophies of contemplation, relaxation, and mind/body connection. From the West he borrowed an emphasis on muscle tone and strength, endurance, and intensity of movement. His method utilizes the whole body, not just a part of it, and Pilates on the Ball should be approached with this key principle in mind. In using the whole body we are balancing the use of the large superficial muscles with the deep, small endurance muscles, those responsible for maintaining a powerful core. This is a very intelligent approach to exercise, an approach that distinguishes this method from many others.

Pilates on the Ball works with what you have. If you are very strong or very weak, injured or in superb shape, a Pilates-based ball session tailored to your needs will be highly beneficial. You should work toward self-education and self-reliance so that you can take away the information you learn in this book and use it to your own benefit.

The deeper you get into the work, and the more you understand its principles, the more the work will be reflected in other parts of your life. Pilates on the Ball is not about compartmentalizing your exercise quota into one or two sessions a week any more than it is about building up some muscle groups and neglecting the rest. Instead this unique ballwork should improve your posture, your back health, your flexibility and overall strength, and your everyday movements in all aspects of your life. Muscle control and postural awareness can translate into how you lift a child, sit in front of a car steering wheel, or hit a tennis ball across a net.

Mind/Body Connection

Pilates on the Ball is mental as well as physical work. The aim is to link the mind with the body. Start by carving out some time for yourself; a silent, uncluttered room will help you focus on the experience. Proper breathing is fundamental to this work and not just tacked on as an afterthought. Proper breathing will help relax you and make the movements feel effortless. The exercises are not introduced as a series of endless repetitions. This is another wonderful aspect of Pilates—no boring repetitions. Joseph Pilates did not believe in overworking the body and neither should you. You will see that the moves are very layered; there is always something new to bring to each move. There is a clear purpose behind each exercise and breathing pattern. Everything in this method is done with precision, focus, and concentration. One makes conscious choices. The mind is very present.

Adding the ball deepens the Pilates experience. The ball will slow things down, heighten your awareness of where your body is in space, and force you to move mindfully. The novelty of the ball's shape plays havoc with your sensation of gravity and mobility and allows you to benefit from nonlinear exploration. The ball will get your attention. Questions will emerge: Where is your body in relationship to the floor? How is your leg rotating in its hip joint? You will start to investigate why you are doing something, what muscles are being used, and how to reeducate those muscles rather than simply going through the motions.

I truly believe that what you give to this ballwork you will get back two- or threefold. The mind/body connection is very powerful and even small conscious moves can be significant and lead to inner shifts. In some movement disciplines, especially those that specialize in body reeducation, thinking through a move can have the same value as physically completing it. The power of the mind can also aid you in changing attitudes and healing the love/hate tug-of-war between inactivity and activity.

At the end of a hard day, instead of collapsing in front of the television, use your ball to do a stretch, calm your mind, and prepare for sleep. Are only two or three stretches worth doing? Of course. Just bring a level of consciousness and commitment to the moves. Playing with your ball may be one of the most pleasurable and soothing gestures your body will ever experience. It could also change your mind and your heart about physical activity forever.

1

A Formidable Partnership

Pilates and the Exercise Ball

Coming Home

When I first laid on a Pilates mat after twenty years of not dancing or doing any sort of physical activity with the exception of walking, surprising and volatile emotions surged up. The first emotion was denial—I don't need this; I have managed for years without structured exercise. Then there was a deep releasing of regret and grief that I could have lived so long without something that felt so soothing and familiar to my body.

During my one-hour session, an experienced Pilates trainer made sure that my shoulders, hips, knees, ankles, and feet were placed in proper alignment. I made sure my emotions were kept in line.

Five days later I tried a second session with another teacher—this time a young apprentice. Good, I thought, a young spandex-clad apprentice with shiny tights and a navel piercing—maybe this time I would be disillusioned.

But the second session was even more profound. This time I knew what was expected and gave the lesson more concentration—just to see what this Pilates work was really all about. Or maybe to kill the sensations that were flooding through my body. "Your body responds well to this," said the young apprentice. Yes, I nodded, afraid to speak.

Twenty years earlier I had walked away from my dream of teaching dance, because I did not believe in myself enough as a dancer to finish my training. Now my hamstrings were stiff. I had very little upper body strength; I had tight hip

[Exercising with a ball] can stir the enthusiast or the slacker, and it can exercise the lower portions of the body or the upper, some particular part rather than the whole . . . or it can exercise all the parts of the body equally . . . [and] is able to give both the most intense workout and the gentlest relaxation.
—Greek philosopher/ physician Galen, second century A.D.

muscles—the results of years of daily long walks without stretching. Yet in spite of my "limitations" (I still judged myself in the language of an old, stern ballet teacher of my past), I instinctively felt the significance and layering of the moves. The young apprentice saw I was hungry to know where the work could go, and she tossed in a couple of intermediate exercises. These involved gentle rolling and tumbling; I giggled inside—this soundless sensation came from a place where the long-lost child gymnast inside of me had been buried for decades.

How had this happened? For twenty years I had avoided my physical self, because I had neatly compartmentalized myself into a mind and a body. From ages twenty to forty I had devoted myself to intellectual pursuits, in particular the relentless struggle to develop a writing career, and I had turned my back on physical endeavors. Alone on the mat after the young apprentice left me to work with someone else, I realized that in choosing a writing career over a physical one, I had lost a part of myself. Pilates, in two mere classes, had not restored it. Nothing could do that. But movement can open people up to a long-forgotten self inside. Dance and movement teachers have often seen this. Curtains are parted, buried dreams surface. Arms stretch heavenward in more ways than one.

I had to pay attention to what these two sessions meant for me. When I stepped off the mat I did feel taller (as the apprentice had promised), but it was a stretching of heart and spirit as much as spine. It was time to shift priorities, and to make room for those changes. It was time to come home.

What Is Pilates—Physiotherapy or Body Conditioning?

During the First World War, German-born Joseph H. Pilates (1880–1967) devised a series of exercises that could overcome injuries and postural problems. Before that he had become an accomplished boxer, gymnast, and circus performer and had personally triumphed over a succession of physical ailments, including asthma and rheumatic fever, by devoting himself to the practice of athletics. Interned in English camps, he began to train other prisoners of war in his matwork exercises. He also devised makeshift exercise aids by attaching bedsprings in various positions so patients recovering from injuries could exercise safely. Modern versions of these pieces of equipment are found in Pilates studios today.

In the late 1920s Joseph Pilates immigrated to New York, bringing his unusual views on physical exercise and fitness with him. Ballet dancers were drawn to his work, investigated its benefits, and began to swear by it. This fact captured my attention when I first heard about the Pilates Method of body conditioning. How could the exercise of choice of back-pain sufferers be challenging enough for a prima ballerina? Why would a series of exercises so closely associated with physical therapy be of any interest to a circus performer or would-be boxer? I imagined a Pilates class to be like a trip to a physical therapy office, except in gym clothes. How wrong I was.

I had, as it turned out, no idea of the scope of the work. The Pilates Method is a complete and thorough program of mental and physical conditioning with an expanding orbit of potential exercises. Many of the small therapeutic movements designed to help people recovering from injuries can be intensified to challenge seasoned athletes. This is what makes the Pilates Method so attractive to the general public, as well as dancers and athletes; it is very versatile work that speaks to all ages and all lev-

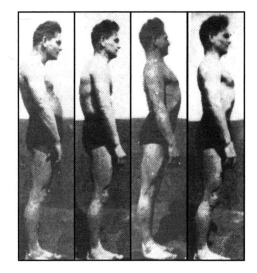

Joseph Pilates, circa 1930, exhibits extremes of various postural tendencies on his way to articulating the ideal, supported posture that is a signature of the Pilates Method. Photographs from Your Health *by Joseph Pilates (1934), currently published by Presentation Dynamics.*

els of fitness. In the past the benefits, which include correcting imbalances, realigning the body, and building core strength from within, were primarily shared by dancers and movie stars. But lately the holistic, preventive-oriented method has been fully embraced by sciatica-plagued carpenters, businesswomen and their physiotherapists, and elite athletes and their sports medicine doctors. As a result the average Pilates teacher sees a vast range of students, many of whom will not set foot in a gym yet are committed to weekly or biweekly group Pilates classes to safely nourish their backs, strengthen their abdominals, and restore elasticity to their bodies.

The Basic Principles of Pilates

Nine principles provide a foundation for how the Pilates Method is organized and executed, and these principles will be discussed throughout the book. First there is *concentration*, the kinesthetic awareness that allows you to focus the mind on what the body is doing. You may need to create a quiet space in order to achieve this level of concentration. You are using the mind to reeducate the muscles, and you should be totally present with the body at all times during this work. Concentration brings with it *control*, the neuromuscular coordination that guarantees movements will not be careless or haphazard. Sometimes our bodies do not perform as we want them to, but coordination and control are skills that can be learned through practice.

Control is achieved by *centering*. Joseph Pilates referred to this as working from a strong core or "girdle of strength." All movement stems outward from the center. Stabilizing from the deep, small core muscles, and the deep as well as superficial abdominals, is a safe and highly effective starting place for movement.

basic principles

The following principles of the Pilates Method are the bedrock on which Pilates on the Ball is built.

Concentration: engaging your mind on what your body is doing

Control: fostering mind/body coordination that guarantees that movements will not be sloppy or haphazard

Centering: working from a strong core

Breathing: breathing into the rib cage

Postural alignment: being aware of the position of your body parts in space

Flow: moving slowly and gracefully

Precision: moving with exact, economic, accurate body-strokes

Stamina: introducing the element of intensity to build endurance when you are ready

Relaxation: learning to release the body and not to overwork it

So is the use of diaphragmatic *breathing*. The breath initiates the movement. Breathing into the back of the rib cage replenishes the body and helps organize the *postural alignment* of the skeleton. If one muscle or bone of the body is out of alignment then the whole structure is affected whether we are sitting on the ball, standing on our feet, or lying on a mat. Faulty alignment negatively affects breath, posture, and movement just as the dominance of one muscle group can affect the quality of movement. The principles of *flow* and *precision* open the door to a holistic movement experience that is as beautiful to watch as it is to perform. Eventually, as we have mastered the exercises, one exact, supple movement will flow into the other. We are aiming for movement that is slow and graceful as well as efficient and accurate.

Finally, and only when you are ready, intensity of movement and the addition of resistance allow *stamina* to be built in the body. We challenge the endurance of the stabilizing muscles without sacrificing form or technique. As important as it is to build up the muscles, it is essential to teach them to relax. *Relaxation* is the key to health and healing of mind and body. A mind/body that knows how to release is a mind/body that will not overwork and overtire. These nine Pilates basic principles are used throughout the Pilates on the Ball Method.

Why Pilates-based Ballwork?

The Pilates Method or Pilates-based work encompasses numerous variations. No two Pilates classes are the same, as many students complain after having participated in a class led by another teacher or located in another city. So why do very few teachers today teach the Pilates Method exactly as it was orginally conceived?

There are various answers. We know much more about the body today, and most leaders in the field of Pilates, even those who studied with Joseph Pilates in the last years of his life, have gone on to devise their own programs and expand the work so that it is safer and more up-to-date. The Canadian expert Moira Stott, who certified me in the Pilates Method, is well respected around the world for her excellent contemporary approach to body conditioning, called Stott Pilates. She trains elite dancers and athletes, but she also has created, without distorting the essence of the work, modifications to make her method highly accessible to ordinary people and those recovering from injuries. Other experts from the world of yoga, dance, the Alexander Technique, and Bartenieff Fundamentals have interpreted the work quite radically but have done so with a keen understanding of its original philosophy and principles. As influential Philadelphia teacher-of-teachers Karen Carlson recently stated at a Pilates Method Workshop in Toronto, it is important to look at the classical legacy of Pilates first before expanding upon it. "Honor the memory of Joseph Pilates," Carlson said, "but use Pilates to better serve the clients."

There is nothing forced or unnatural about adapting Pilates to the ball. Both have had a close association with physiotherapy: like the Pilates Method, Pilates on the Ball is primarily concerned with aligning the body, isolating and training deep postural muscles, and building torso strength without reinjuring or harming the body. With the ball you can isolate a body part if you need to, for example, to rehabilitate a knee or a shoulder. However, the ball also teaches you to work with the torso as a whole—a key principle in the Pilates Method. Other inherent Pilates principles adapt smoothly to the ball and will be discussed throughout this book. Concepts such as centering or "navel-to spine" are crucial when we climb on the ball, which is an unstable base of support. Fluidity of movement and refinement of the mind/body connection can be enhanced by working with the ball, because it allows the user to experience the reaction of the movement on the entire body. Relaxation and breathing are vital components to a Pilates workout, and the ball is an excellent tool to enhance relaxation and guide the breath into the right place in the body.

Combining the principles, exercises, and breathing patterns of the Pilates Method with the dynamic qualities of the exercise ball creates wonderful results. But to appreciate the full repercussions of those results it is important to look at the unique benefits that the exercise ball delivers to any workout.

The Unique Power of the Ball

The exercise ball is light, portable, durable, and inexpensive. Unlike any other piece of equipment or a mat, the ball is an unstable base of support. Pitting your gravity-bound body against a mobile ball requires balance, and balancing recruits many of the body's deep, stabilizing muscles. Most of these muscles are underused, resulting in the most common injuries of the knee, ankle, shoulder, or back.

Ed McNeely, the man who created the fitness regime for the Canadian gold-medal-winning Olympic rowing team, told the Toronto *Globe and Mail* newspaper that the exercise ball, sometimes called the Swiss ball, was his workout of choice. He stated that "with a Swiss ball you are stabilizing muscles and working deeper layers of muscles, and working them in a way that is more functional." Exercise machines support the back and buttocks, which often means that these areas relax during a workout and are not recruited. On the ball, muscles must keep working.

At the same time it is strengthening the body, the exercise ball heightens proprioception—your awareness of how your body moves in space. The ball helps focus your attention on how you perceive and interpret stimuli and sensations from the world around you. This is how the ball is used to rehabilitate motor skills, increase sensory perception, and intensify athletic performance. By increasing the speed of the workout or narrowing the base of support, more challenge is added. This helps elite athletes kick, swing, and jump with more control and power.

The ball allows you to practice falling with safety and grace. These skills are significant as we age. Physical therapist and exercise ball pioneer Joanne Posner-Mayer explains that individuals with poor balance fear and avoid activities where balance is further compromised or challenged. This creates a cycle in which fear leads to further inactivity. Athletes, as well as ordinary people, will benefit enormously from practicing balance and recovery skills.

The postural muscles, which are close to the vertebral column, maintain an erect spine. Bad posture rounds the back, compresses the lungs, and causes these deep spinal muscles to become "deprogrammed," or weak. In contrast,

Short History of the Exercise Ball

nicknamed the "Swiss ball" by North American therapists who saw the balls in use in the 1960s in Switzerland, these large 55- or 65-cm balls were initially employed in Europe for the treatment of orthopedic problems, for increasing somatic awareness, and for encouraging pediatric neurological development. Manufactured in 1963 in Italy by Aquilino Cosani, an Italian toy maker, the vinyl balls were first sold to physical therapists, hospitals, and clinics. According to American physical therapist Joanne Posner-Mayer, the history of the exercise ball as a therapy tool probably begins with the Swiss pediatrician Dr. Elsbeth Köng. In the late 1950s Köng and Mary Quinton, an English physiotherapist, worked with physically challenged children using the Bobath Method of neuromuscular reeducation.

In the 1970s Joanne Posner-Mayer completed her Bobath training in Switzerland with Köng and Quinton, and worked with therapists trained by ball specialists Dr. Susanne Klein-Vogelbach and the Czech physical therapist

Maria Kucera. Klein-Vogelbach has been particularly influential in theory, exercises, and clinical applications of the ball, and was the first to use balls on adult orthopedic patients. Her book *Ball Gymnastik for Functional Kinetics* was published in 1980 in Germany.

In 1995, based on twenty years of experience, Posner-Mayer wrote the manual *Swiss Ball Applications for Orthopedic and Sports Medicine*. Posner-Mayer is concerned with injury prevention and wellness but she also realizes that the ball is beneficial for healthy individuals. In 1998 a German-born physical therapist and student of Klein-Vogelbach, Beate Carrière, wrote an extensive textbook for physical therapists. *The Swiss Ball: Theory, Basic Exercises, and Clinical Application* focuses on a wide range of treatments in all areas of physical therapy, including gynecologic disorders. Recently the ball has moved out of the exclusive realm of physical therapy and is now used in elite training and general fitness applications.

sitting on the ball is highly advantageous for back health because it is active work: the body continually adjusts to maintain balance. Over time, ball sitting retrains postural muscles and brings the body back into balance.

Bouncing on the ball creates a dynamic, yet safe, cardiovascular workout that will protect your heart and lungs. Moreover, the ball cushions your body as you bounce, at the same time training the feet to safely absorb the impact of landing. Posner-Mayer attests that by continually moving the feet the base of support is reduced and the center of gravity changes. This forces the body to make constant adjustments to maintain balance. The abdominal muscles work too: if you slouch on the ball, or let go of your abdominals, you will soon discover that the ball will drift. Plus, bouncing on the ball burns calories!

Another significant advantage of the ball is the addition of resistance and weight-bearing: this is what attracted my attention when I first decided to integrate the ball with the matwork. Lifting the ball in the air with the arms, or the legs, adds resistance. Taking weight on your hands or your feet while your body partially rests on the ball adds weight-bearing. Moreover, placing the hands or feet on the ground fosters a direct connection with the ground that teaches us to process the environment around our bodies as well as the movement of our bodies.

Nowhere can the degree of weight transfer be better practiced than on a mobile ball, which is precisely why the exercise ball is used in so many elite training centers throughout the world. When we lift one leg or one arm we cause a shift in weight, and a rapid adjustment must be made in the body. Working upper and lower torso, or oppositionally—one side of the body and then the other—requires the simultaneous participation of the entire body and quick and flexible motor control.

Finally, the most exceptional features that the ball offers are its shape and texture. Light and filled with air, the ball provides a comfortable but firm surface that uniquely supports the user in varying positions in space. The ball's extraordinary potential for three-dimensional exploration is eloquently described by Dr. Ninoska Gomez in her *Somarhythms* video: "The force of gravity becomes a challenging partner when you realize that sensing and moving the body's weight is playful, risky, and creative." It is impossible to stretch or open the body with a mat or a machine in the way that can be achieved with a spherical, air-filled ball.

Other Uses for the Ball

Physiotherapists are recommending replacing chairs with balls in schools throughout Europe. Teachers found that hyperactive children could focus for longer periods and most children could generally concentrate better and

ninoska gomez's somarhythms ballwork

Dr. Gomez is a developmental psychologist and movement instructor in Canada and Latin America. In her short video, *Somarhythms* (see Resources on page 170), she explores somatic awareness and space relations through rolling, falling, balancing, gliding, pushing, pulling, and bouncing with large balls. In the video she explores the texture of the ball on the face, cheek, forehead, chin, forearm, and palms as well as other parts of the body.

develop a superior sense of organization sitting on a ball rather than a chair. Studies are now being conducted to test the impact of ball sitting on children with attention deficient disorder (ADD).

The ball is fantastic for de-stressing and stretching. Massage and other bodywork therapists use small and large balls to teach their clients to stretch out their problem areas and release the body from harmful tensions. For example, Yamuna Zake, creator of Body Rolling, uses eight- to twelve-inch balls to elongate muscles, release tension, and create space in the body. Some find that the ball helps bring to the surface old emotional wounds.

Other therapists have been creatively introducing the ball to various movement disciplines. Mari Naumovski, a Toronto-based movement therapist and certified Pilates instructor who brings a Laban/Bartenieff approach to the exercise ball, has developed a system called BodySpheres. She focuses on the two unique features of the ball: shape and texture. "We use our whole body in relation to the ball, as if the ball is a partner or an extension of our own body," explains Naumovski, adding: "the ball enhances breath connection, three-dimensional movement, interchange of mobility and stability, and sequencing." (See box below.)

Yoga practitioners are now employing balls to facilitate relaxation and to enable students to achieve postures that they would never accomplish without the ball as an aid. Continuum and other somatic systems use large balls in exploring breath and sound. Balls are also used as therapy for strengthening pelvic-floor muscles and treating incontinence, as well as preparing for childbirth and healing nerve injuries sustained during delivery.

Mari Naumovski's BodySpheres

*b*odySpheres, invented by Canadian movement therapist Mari Naumovski, is an approach to exercise, body awareness, and three-dimensional exploration that uses 45- to 65-cm balls. Mari works with balls that are slightly underinflated so there is more responsiveness to changes in body weight.

Pilates ballwork focuses on core strength. Naumovski's BodySpheres expands on the precise control of the Pilates Method to incorporate circular/spherical movements and rotations in different planes. Listen to some of the wonderful names of her exercises: Cat Nudging, Baby Tailbone Rolls, Sandwich Stretch, and Leap Frog, to name a few. Each shows a playful approach to ballwork. However, there is also an inherent sophistication to her work; she is interested in the overall physical organization of body connections, and many of her body positions provide abundant sensory and motor stimulation.

With Mari's permission I've included three of her unique exercises in this book.

Before You Start

Before you embrace the unique partnership of the Pilates Method and the exercise ball, please consider some general guidelines. As with any form of mind/body conditioning, you must concentrate and focus to get the full benefits of this work. Sometimes this means first learning the exercises without the ball. Unless you have had substantial Pilates training, you will want to start with one exercise at a time. Read through all the instructions before you attempt an exercise, and pay attention to the watchpoints and modifications. I present variations throughout the book, and it is important to master these before you work up to more challenging versions. Remember that there may be days when, out of the blue, you have neck strain or lower back pain and you will want to utilize the modification so you can keep your body moving in spite of the pain. I have found that even accomplished athletes, usually because of tightness in the hips or hamstrings, are sometimes unable to master a full exercise. At times an exercise may require coordination or control that is still unfamiliar to you. If you are not fit or are recovering from an injury, you will have to work up to the full version gradually. Even if physical constraints prevent you from doing the full versions, you will still be able to attain benefits. Remember that just sitting on the ball is an endurance activity and is therefore beneficial; but whether sitting or bouncing, start slow and build.

When you are ready for the advanced work, by all means add it to your routine. Be careful not to add too much too soon. Because of the shape of the ball you may experience a fuller range of motion than you are used to; a slight soreness may result. Working on a mobile ball will tax you in new ways. You may fatigue more quickly as muscles that are rarely challenged get a unique workout.

Occasionally I have students who have trouble in the beginning adjusting to the demands of the ball. Perseverance pays off. Slow things down; visualize what you are trying to accomplish with each move. Practice gives you the skills: each time it will get easier. Another possible discomfort is motion sickness. A small percentage of students experience motion sickness when using the ball. It is generally only two or three moves from the entire repertoire that bring this on, and I have noted them. If you feel the onset of motion sickness, stop, and take some deep breaths. Immediately make note of which exercise brought on the sensation. Alter this exercise to be a much smaller movement or omit it completely.

Choose the exercises that grab you but also pay attention to those that you instinctively turn away from. Sometimes we resist the exercises that we need the most. Watchpoints, by the way, are not meant to be a critical

15

voice. They are simply hints to help you perform the exercise better. We are recovering movement, not censoring it.

The Right Ball for You

Exercise balls are inexpensive and widely available in health and fitness shops. Be warned: all balls are not created equal. Some are cheap to the touch and to the smell. I personally prefer Fitball (see page 171 for ordering information). I love these pearl- or black-colored balls because they have an excellent surface that is not dangerously slippery. They are also burst resistant: if you accidentally roll over a sharp object they will not explode but deflate gradually. Fitballs even have a faint pleasant vanilla aroma, not a strong vinyl smell. They are weight tested to 1,000 pounds for normal use.

The appropriate size of the ball is a subject of debate among teachers and depends on what exercise method you will be using. I find that with Pilates-based work the 55-cm ball is perfect unless you are very tall (and strong). The larger the ball, the heavier and more unwieldy it is. A general rule is that when sitting on the ball the hips and knees should be bent at a 90-degree angle. This usually translates to 55 cm for people 5' to 5'8" and 65 cm for 5'8" to 6'2".

Balls are blown up according to diameter, not air pressure. A yardstick will help you inflate to maximum diameter (height off the floor), which is printed on the ball and on the box. Only inflate to the recommended diameter and not bigger. Fitballs come with long plugs that cannot be swallowed by children, and these plugs are very easy to put in and take out of the ball for travel. Use an air raft or mattress pump or go to a gas station and use a cone-shaped trigger nozzle. Most people find that a bicycle pump is simply not forceful enough. Most exercise ball distributors offer a small, inexpensive, plastic pump that is totally portable and very effective for inflating the ball in one or two minutes.

Some simple precautions will help you care for your ball.

- Do not use the ball outside, and do not let children (or animals) use the ball.
- Keep your ball out of direct sunlight and away from direct heat sources.
- Most balls clean up quickly with a cloth and warm soapy water.

This Is Your Ride

Before you start your Pilates on the Ball work, let's review some helpful hints and precautions:

- Check with your doctor or health care practitioner to be sure these exercises are suitable for you. Pay attention to modifications and stop if there is any discomfort. If in doubt, avoid an exercise.
- A "less is more" approach applies to this method as it does to so much else in life where wisdom prevails. If you have pain, you are pushing yourself too hard.
- With any exercise routine it is not advisable to exercise after a meal. This is especially so with Pilates on the Ball.
- Start gradually. Be sure you have drinking water handy.
- Bare feet connect best with the floor. If you still find your feet slipping, use rubber-soled shoes.
- Work on a sticky yoga mat or a slip-resistant rug.
- Be sure to have plenty of space around you.
- If clothing or long hair is loose, it can get caught under the ball.
- Check that the area is clear of staples, small stones, or other objects that may damage the ball.
- Work in two or three sessions a week. If you prefer short sessions daily, combine moves that focus on strength with moves that focus on stretching.

One of the best aspects of Pilates on the Ball is that most students report immediate results. Even after one session they feel taller and lighter, and so will you. After a few sessions you will marvel as your abdominals become stronger and your posture becomes easier and more upright. Suddenly you will enjoy performing an exercise, like push-ups, for example, which you never thought you would do again in your life. You may notice a change in the shape of your arms, as this area is usually weak, especially in women: the arms are one of the first places where you will see visible results. You may notice that the philosophies learned in this book are radiating into other aspects of your life: suddenly you may become aware that you have slouched for too long in front of a desk without rewarding your body with a stretch.

Only you are in control of your fitness level and the lifestyle choices that you make. Combining the dynamic functions of the exercise ball with the principles and philosophies of the Pilates Method can change your quality of life and your back health, but only if you can strike a balance between accomplishment and challenge.

2

Breathing and Breathers

Joseph Pilates's Story

A young boy growing up near Dussledorf, Germany, in the late 1800s dreams of boxing and a life as a circus performer. Instead, he is often sick, even confined to his bed, and his breathing takes on a jagged wheeze as it struggles in and out of his young body. One morning he wakes up in a sweat and feels pain in his elbows and wrists. His parents fear another grim bout with childhood rickets, but this time it is rheumatic fever that sets him back. When he recovers he propels himself into physical activity, eventually taking up bodybuilding as if to defy his sickly body. He has a gift for gymnastics but sometimes has to quit when his chest tightens and he coughs up phlegm. He experiments with muscle control and learns how to make his movements more efficient. He desires total fitness, and everyone around him notices his well-developed physique. If only he could achieve a full breath.

This German youth had taught his body new boxing, diving, and tumbling moves. Why not discipline it to breathe correctly? He knew his ability to exhale was diminished by his asthma so he worked at squeezing every bit of air from his lungs. Placing his hands on his rib cage, he focused on the exhale. He discovered that totally freeing the lungs of air created a vacuum, which allowed the lungs to refill naturally with air. Still, freeing the rib cage was harder to achieve than he thought. Sometimes he inhaled more deeply than he was used to, and he felt lightheaded. His goal was to draw in the abdomen, expand the chest and rib cage to capacity, and be sure that the exhale was sufficient to deflate the lungs properly. It made perfect sense. The secret to correct breathing lies in the diaphragm.

Diaphragmatic breathing became a crucial component of this athlete's evolving conditioning program. One day his exercises, eventually to be known as the Pilates Method, would become famous and transform the way dancers, athletes, physiotherapists, and the general exercising population view movement and exercise.

Back Breathing

When we breathe well we create the optimum conditions for health and can feel its positive influence on all aspects of our being. As Joseph Pilates discovered, too often we do not breathe properly and only use a fraction of our lung capacity. As babies we employed deep belly-breathing and effective diaphragmatic breathing to comfort and relax us. How did we grow up to become labored breathers and chest lifters?

The famous fight-or-flight response—the primitive protective instinct brought on by extreme stress—causes hyperventilation or shallow rapid breathing in modern humans, even though we have no beast or foe to fight off physically. This superficial breathing causes tension to accumulate in the upper body, the neck, between the shoulder blades, and even in the jaw and facial muscles. More alarming, a number of significant studies show that incorrect breathing correlates with heart palpitations and chest pains and that there is a link between people who display incorrect breathing characteristics and the risk of coronary heart disease.

It was because Joseph Pilates was an asthma sufferer that he discovered the power of diaphragmatic breathing—of sending the breath into the rib cage. He spoke of "squeezing every atom of pure air from your lungs," the importance of a full inhalation and full exhalation. It is not known how Pilates's diaphragmatic breathing affects conditions such as asthma and emphysema, yet some of my students who previously gasped and gulped for air have told me how after a Pilates class their asthmatic wheeze is gone. One student, a fifty-five-year-old woman, remarked: "I feel entirely different after class. I feel energized. My breathing channels feel that they are open, whereas before class they were restricted, tighter. I can take a deep breath as a result of the class, whereas I could not take a deep breath before." Pilates trainer-to-the-stars and asthma sufferer Mari Winsor attests how Pilates breathing helped relieve her wheezing, and it has been a long time since she has had a full-blown asthma attack.

The diaphragm is a dome-shaped muscular wall between the chest and the abdominals. It is designed to work like a pump; on the in breath it contracts and moves downward, drawing in air as the rib cage opens. On the out breath the diaphragm relaxes and the dome rises, discharging used air.

Without restrictions the diaphragm not only moves up and down but also billows outward.

In Pilates on the Ball we try to guide the breath not into the abdominals or the upper chest, but into the lower rib cage. This is called back breathing. Back breathing utilizes the full spectrum of breathing muscles: the thoracic, intercostal (rib cage), and back muscles, as well as the deep transversus abdominal and oblique muscles that contract the abdominal area. Think of expanding the rib cage sideways, as well as forward and backward. As we attempt three-dimensional breathing we do not want to restrict the natural ballooning of the belly. Chronic tight contraction of the abdominals pulls down on the lower ribs, interferes with the pumplike downward motion of the diaphragm, and causes superficial chest breathing. However, when we start to move from the abdominal center or inner core of support called the power-house, we need to be sure that the lower back is protected. We do this by ensuring that the abdominals are fully engaged as we perform the exercises.

Breathing Patterns as Therapy

Correct breathing nurtures the body and releases toxins. On the inhale, oxygen travels to the cells, purifies the bloodstream, and nourishes the muscles. On the exhale, unused gases stored in the body are expelled. The breath, when used correctly, is a very powerful force in the body for soothing nervous tension, improving concentration, and directly controlling energy levels.

Like any other muscle in the body, respiratory muscles can have poor tone. In Pilates on the Ball, breathing is a key principle: we attempt to teach the entire respiratory system to breathe efficiently. The breath is a starting point for each exercise and there is a breathing pattern to accompany each exercise. These patterns are flexible and can be altered to each student's needs and limitations. For example, some students find that inhaling while performing a certain movement causes them to lift the shoulders to the ears rather than what is required—a sliding down of the shoulder blades. An exhalation for this movement may work better for some students. The general rule is to inhale to prepare and exhale to exert. We strive for natural breathing, not forced or controlled breathing. Above all, do not hold your breath.

The Pilates breathing patterns are therapy in themselves. We attempt to slow down the breath, increase the depth of respiration, and link the breath to the movement. Remember that we want a complete inhalation as well as a complete exhalation. The out breath should be as full as possible. Of primary importance is removing the effort from breathing: we want to reduce the work of the respiratory muscles, not increase it. Often students try too hard in the beginning and force the inhalation so that they become dizzy or light-headed. This usually goes away with practice. Remember that it is not necessary to force the inhalation, because when the exhalation is complete and the air is totally emptied from the lungs, a vacuum will be created and the air will be sucked back naturally into the lungs.

The breathing patterns help us blend one movement into the next. Pilates on the Ball is very mindful work; we are moving the body in a very specific way, and the breathing cues us from one movement to the next. At first marrying the breath with the movement may feel difficult. Persevere but don't force. Try less movement. Even less breath. Try and find the bottom of the exhale—that moment of peace and calm before the action of the inhale. This choreographed breathing helps relax muscles and relieve tension in the body and utilizes the mind as well as the body. It also safeguards us from holding our breath.

The Breathing Exercises

Back breathing, or rib cage breathing, takes time to master. When I was completing my Pilates training, I found the breathing one of the most challenging parts of my extensive course. Some of the trainees had trouble linking breath with movement; I had trouble getting the breath in the right place, especially when I added movements. Even on a visit to an observant physiotherapist, where I was laying on a table doing nothing, I was reminded that I was still breathing incorrectly! Do not be discouraged if you can't master the breathing at once. Fear or shame that you are not performing well, not doing the breathing correctly, can ruin the experience and increase tension in the muscles. It can also cause that which we want least: breath holding.

The ball is a wonderful tool, because it will help you actually see and physically feel how the breath can be channeled into different parts of the body. The ball will help those who know too little about anatomy, or too much. Forget all that you know and imagine the ball as your lungs! Or feel the breath initiating from different parts of the body: the pelvis, the bottoms of the feet, anywhere that will allow a full-body experience of the breath. In the following three breathing exercises—Observations, Back Breathing, and Side Breathing—your body will be in a different relationship to gravity, and you will feel the breath differently because of this. Take time with these exercises. Remember how Joseph Pilates used the lengthening of the exhalation as a way of getting to the inhale. Try it yourself. Take a moment to discover the pleasure and health of a well-rounded breath.

The rib cage is not fixed but is instead a very mobile interplay of living malleable tissue.
—Frank Bach,
Conscious Movement
Workshop

21

Breathing Observations

In this exercise you will explore how the breath can be directed easily into different parts of the body. The ball isolates the front of the body, and this will aid you in feeling the difference between abdominal breathing and rib cage or back breathing. As you attempt these two observations visualize your spine lengthening in two opposing directions: out from the tailbone and up each vertebra through the crown of your head. In movement 1 try placing a gentle pressure of the hands on the top of the ball to give the breathing muscles something to resist against. Keep nostrils open and relaxed. We are inhaling through the nose and exhaling through the mouth with a relaxed jaw.

Purpose To direct the breath into different parts of the body.

Watchpoints • Keep the body loose and relaxed. • Inhale through the nose, exhale through the mouth. • The ball will barely move during rib cage breathing, though you may feel the movement in your hands as the lungs open and contract. • Notice how much more the ball lifts on the abdominal observations.

starting position

1. Lie on your back with your knees bent and your feet hip-distance apart.
2. Place the ball on your chest.

movement 1: abdominal breathing

1. Roll the ball down to your belly. Be sure that the feet are not too close to the buttocks so that the ball can rest squarely on your abdomen (fig. 2.1).
2. Inhale through the nose to fill the abdominals with air.
3. Exhale to empty the air fully from the belly.
4. Take five deep breaths in this manner.
5. Notice that the ball gently lifts as the abdominals balloon and drops as the abdominals flatten.

movement 2: rib cage or back breathing

1. Roll the ball up to the point where the sternum ends and the rib cage opens (fig. 2.2).
2. Inhale to fill the back of the rib cage with breath.
3. Exhale to close the front of the body.
4. Take five deep breaths into the rib cage in this manner.

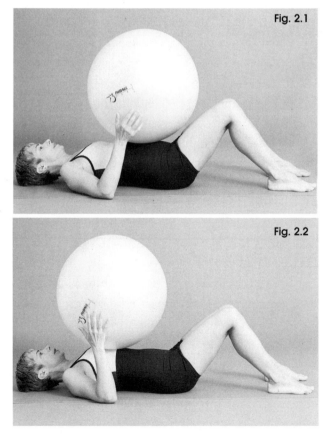

Fig. 2.1

Fig. 2.2

Back Breathing

Back breathing is another term for rib cage breathing. The Shell or Child's pose is a perfect position to direct the breath into the back space of the rib cage. You will feel a wonderful elongation through the sacral, lumbar, and middle spine. The arms extended on the ball add a deep stretch to the neck and arms. Avoid this exercise if you have knee problems; try the modification instead. Think of a fish breathing through its gills.

Purpose To practice breathing into the back rib cage. To stretch the spine, arms, and neck.

Watchpoints • Concentrate on sending your breath into the back rib cage without causing tension in any part of the body. • You may need a cushion under your ankles to get comfortable in the Shell position. • If your knees feel even a slight strain, place a cushion between your buttocks and your knees. • Avoid the Shell if you have knee problems. Use the modification instead.

Modification If the Shell stretch is too hard on your body, open your legs, set the ball between the legs, and hug the ball. Follow the movement instructions, taking five breaths, slow and deep.

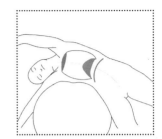

three-dimensional breathing on the ball

The diaphragm, a dome-shaped muscle wall between the chest and the abdominals, is the primary muscle of respiration. It is designed not only to move up and down but also to billow sideways.

Use your ball as a tool to help you focus on sending the breath into the rib cage. Think of expanding the rib cage sideways as well as forward and backward. Do not force the inhalation; a full exhalation creates a vacuum and air will be sucked back naturally into the lungs. Whatever you do, do not hold your breath.

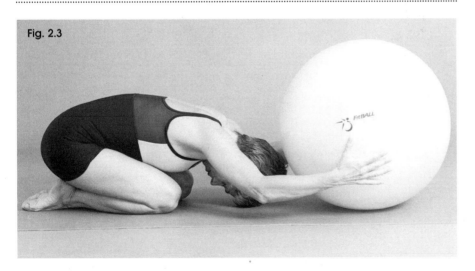

Fig. 2.3

starting position

Kneel on a rug or a mat. Extend your arms long in front of you, hands on the outside of the ball (fig. 2.3).

movement

1. Slowly sit back on your heels, rounding your back and relaxing your neck.

2. Inhale through your nose to expand the back of the rib cage.
3. Exhale through your mouth to release.
4. Take five breaths, slow and deep, in this manner.

Side Breathing

Here we are working to direct the breath into the side rib cage. Lying over the ball on your right side presses the right rib cage against the ball so that the air is forced into the left rib cage. You will feel a stretch and an opening up of the left side of the body.

Purpose To direct the breath into the side rib cage as well as the back rib cage.

Watchpoints • Be sure that you have enough free space around you in case you lose your balance. • If you experience neck or arm strain, support your head with your hand and drop your overhead arm onto the ball. • Focus the breath into the rib cage without creating tension in the neck, shoulders, or upper chest.

Modification If you have knee problems push into the outstretched foot and try to get the weight off the bent knee. Be careful not to lose your balance.

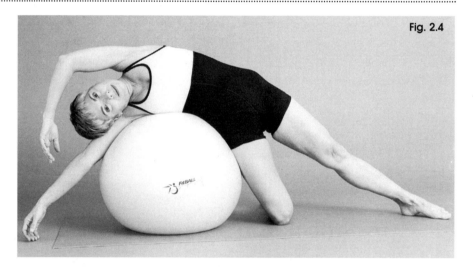

Fig. 2.4

starting position

1. Kneel upright next to your ball so that the right side of your body is close to the ball.

2. Keep your right knee bent as you straighten out your left leg to the side, hands on the ball.

movement

1. Carefully shift your weight to the right side and allow the right side of the body to relax over the ball, left arm stretching overhead. Your head can rest on the right shoulder if this is comfortable (fig. 2.4).

2. Inhale into the left rib cage.

3. Exhale to release.

4. Take five breaths in this manner and then slowly come out of the stretch.

5. Before moving to the left side, see if you can sense more expansion in the opened-up left side of the rib cage and waist.

6. Repeat this movement sequence on the left side.

Breathers—Cocoons of Readiness

A "breather" is a release from effort and strain. Breathers are as important in your workout as they are in daily life. It is crucial that we learn to release the body from tension and negative self-images and calm the conscious mind so that everyday traumas will not transfer to and harm the body. As faulty breathing habits become a permanent state of being, our bodies can be constantly agitated, on guard to fight for survival—a response to modern stress. Our very health depends on learning how to let the body unwind and recharge.

In Pilates on the Ball we do not want to overwork the body. This is why there are relaxation positions built in to the workout. Think of these as states of cocooning: we are relaxed, yet ready. We slow down and scan the body before each exercise to be sure that we are in the correct position and that we are not holding tension. If so, we can release that particular area, whether it be the back of the neck, the shoulders, or a rigid hand gripping the side of the mat. We focus the mind on how we transform the body. And when we do move, our movement assumes the powerful quality of metamorphosis. Our metamorphosis is initiated by breath, with only the precise amount of exertion that is necessary. Overworking the body can cause injuries. It also creates exhaustion, diminishing results, and rigidity of the mind and body.

Breathe . . .

*R*emember to practice the breathing exercises from time to time. Next time you feel stress, restlessness, or anxiety take over your body, reach for your ball, and breathe. Each inhale should energize and center you. Each exhale should drain out soreness and tension and plunge you into a deep pool of calm. Try it. Right now—one long breath out. Do you feel more relaxed?

Keep your ball in a convenient location. Devote a space where you can use it and get into the habit of reaching for it to restore equilibrium after a stressful day, just as you would slip into a soothing bath. Some students report that just looking at their ball fosters release and relaxation. Even people who have trouble relaxing in yoga or meditation class acknowledge that the ball helps their bodies release.

This chapter introduces you to the crucial starting point for all this work—the breath. Sometimes people feel that "just lying around breathing" can't be challenging. Or since all of us breathe every day and have as much practice as our lives are long, it may appear strange that we must spend an entire chapter on relearning how to breathe. If you are tempted to skip over this chapter, you will miss the greatest benefits of Pilates on the Ball. In fact, you will want to review this chapter as your expertise progresses.

The following three breathers are key transitional positions used throughout the Pilates on the Ball workout. These poses can be used on their own for relaxation or as tranquil positions to practice breathing. These positions, as well as all transitions, are as important as the exercises themselves. As soon as you learn the exercises you will begin to achieve the sense of flow that is so essential to this work. Remember, a breather is not an opportunity to let everything go and sprawl in exhaustion on your mat. It is a chance to release muscular tension and allow your joints to decompress while remaining in correct alignment. It is also an opportunity to focus and concentrate on the next move.

Breather One

Often lying flat on the back with your legs straight is uncomfortable, especially if you have any lower back pain or discomfort. Slipping the ball under your knees releases the lower back from undue stress. A small flat pillow under the head may make you more comfortable. If your feet are cold, wear socks. Have a blanket nearby. Let the breath work with you to erase the traumas of the day.

Purpose To relax body and mind.
Watchpoints • Do not rush into relaxation. • Scan the body and notice where you are holding tension or discomfort. • Rib cage or belly breathing is fine during all of the Breathers.

starting position
Lie flat on your back on a rug or a mat with the legs up on the ball (fig. 2.5).

movement
1. Allow your eyelids to close. Focus on your breath, especially on the long exhale and the overall feeling of ease that it brings to the body.
2. Take a series of deep, slow breaths.

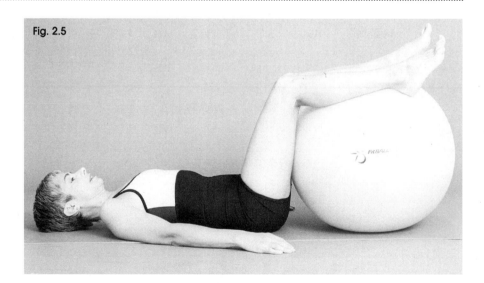
Fig. 2.5

Breather Two

A variation on yoga's Little Boat pose, this position is often used as a link between one move and another. Hold the ball on your shins or knees but use as little effort as possible. Keep the back of the neck long. Let the lower back relax onto the mat; if you want you can add a small rocking motion from side to side.

Purpose To release the lower back and groin. To stretch the back of the thighs.
Watchpoints • Be sure that the back of the neck is released when the head is on the mat. • You may need to gently drop the chin, as if you are holding a tennis ball at your throat.

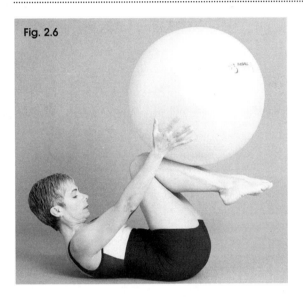

Fig. 2.6

starting position

Lie on your back. Bend your knees into your chest and place the ball on the shins or knees.

movement

1. Inhale to prepare.
2. Exhale to gently pull the ball closer, drawing the knees in deeper. Rock a little from side to side.
3. Hug the knees closer and lift your head for two counts (fig. 2.6). Then lower your head to the mat.

Breather Three

If you have worked with your ball a bit and have grown accustomed to it, you can try lying over the ball. This relaxation pose is different from the other two. You will not be able to hold it for a long time, as you are balancing on your hands and feet. (Do not attempt this on a full stomach.) Most people love this pose: not only does it open up the upper spine and release the neck muscles, but it gives one the sensation of womblike safety and comfort. Occasionally I have come across a student who feels nausea or motion sickness when he or she rolls over the ball and brushes the head inches from the mat. For those students I suggest that they kneel before the ball, bring one knee in and then the other, and hug the ball, releasing the head to one side.

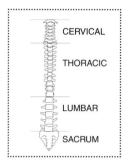

CERVICAL

THORACIC

LUMBAR

SACRUM

anatomy on the ball: the spine

As you allow your spine to take the shape of the ball, imagine in your mind's eye your backbone. Your spine consists of twenty-four spool-shaped vertebrae plus the sacrum—the triangular bone at the base of the spine. Below the sacrum is your tailbone.

As gravity gently opens you up and you feel a pleasant release in the neck and upper spine, can you image the sections of the spine? In the cervical section there are seven neck bones, or vertebrae; in the thoracic, or upper back, there are twelve; and in the lumbar, or lower back, there are five.

Because of the number of bones that make up the spine, and the joints between them, the spine is very mobile. Go deeper into your stretch, so that your head is one inch from the ground. Send the breath into your back. Allow gravity to do its work. Enjoy!

Purpose To relax body and mind. To allow gravity to naturally stretch the neck and spine.

Watchpoints • Take care that long hair does not get stuck under the ball as you roll forward. • The chest and breasts should not feel compressed. Letting a small amount of air out of the ball makes this pose more comfortable for some.

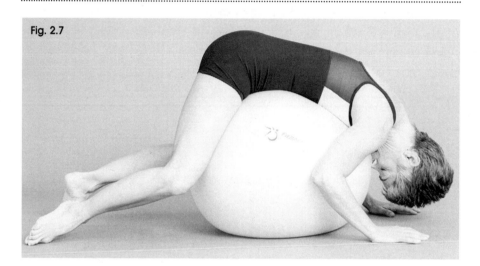

Fig. 2.7

starting position
Kneel behind the ball and carefully lay your body over it, face down.

movement
1. Keeping the movement small to begin, roll over the ball, face down.

2. Place your hands a few inches apart on the ground in front of the ball, toes on the ground behind you.
3. Go deeper into the stretch so that your head is only one inch from the ground (fig. 2.7).

4. Feel your spine release.
5. Practice breathing into the back of the rib cage. Then try breathing deep into the abdominals, noticing how the pelvic muscles release with that breath.

Rib cage breathing takes time to master but the results are well worth the effort. Return to this chapter from time to time and review the breathing exercises. It is important to remember that the breathing patterns in the following chapters are not written in stone. Many teachers and students take liberties with breathing patterns and so can you. The most important thing is not to hold your breath. Be sure that you build breathers or relaxation positions into your workout. In the next chapter we will begin to add body movements to the breath patterns. The postural exercises are designed to foster an awareness of your spine. Sitting, bouncing, and performing the postural exercises will strengthen the deep small spinal muscles and bring the body back into balance.

3
The Postural Exercises

Elsie's Story

Elsie is a statuesque eighty-something-year-old woman who appears to be sixty, maybe even younger. A life of pampering and wealth? No. She grew up during the Depression, the third oldest child in a poverty-stricken family of six girls raised by her mother as her father labored in the mines. The family survived on the food they grew themselves, and Elsie's early mornings were spent hauling firewood and feeding the goat and chickens. Like many who grew up poor, Elsie endured numerous disappointments. She was a talented basketball player, but when her unimaginable dream came true and her local team, the Edmonton Grads, qualified for the 1936 Olympics in Berlin, Germany, Elsie could not accompany them. Her family couldn't afford the uniforms or travel expenses, and Elsie watched from afar as, without her, her team won the gold medal. Life threw many other curveballs in her path, including a very difficult marriage that pulled her in a thousand directions in her role as mother and wife. There were times when she was hurting and times when she sent blessings into the world. Through it all she kept her head up.

When I first met Elsie I was immediately struck by her youthfulness even though she was my oldest student. She had the air of a socialite and the walk of a dancer. She did not let her aging body hang like a tired sack over her long bones. Her excellent posture sculpted decades from her appearance and put many of my twenty-one-year-old students to shame. Her face was lined, but her carriage was regal. Elsie's posture was her beauty secret.

Postural Types

Poor posture does more than diminish the appearance of self-confidence and dignity: it hampers proper breathing, strains muscles and ligaments, and can adversely affect the joints of the back, which are prone to arthritis, sciatica, and generalized pain. The vulture-shaped neckline of a kyphotic posture—head projected forward and scooped shoulders—chronically pulls on the muscles in the neck. Sometimes accompanying kyphosis is a lordosis posture, an exaggerated curve in the lower back that can cause the lower vertebral disks to be squeezed or pinched, causing pain. Swayback posture, another common alignment problem, is caused by a pelvis that has moved forward of where it should be, resulting in a slumped appearance.

Compared to these examples, you may imagine your postural problems are small, yet intelligible. Perhaps you have felt how a hip or a knee can lock in one position so that standing is painful or tiring. Or maybe you have noticed signs of wear-and-tear on one side of your shoes, an indication of faulty weight shift in your gait. Perhaps a health care practitioner has told you that you have a C- or S-shape spine. A lateral curvature of the spine is called scoliosis and is more common than you might think.

Poor posture may be a result of structural problems, muscular imbalances, or simply bad habits. We have inherited different body shapes and tendencies and these cannot be changed overnight. However, the Pilates Method is known to be highly effective in realigning the body and addressing postural weaknesses by targeting the small postural muscles on both sides of the spine. The ball exercises in this chapter live up to this claim. Depending on the severity of the scoliosis, Pilates on the Ball will help most mild cases by creating mobility and space in the back, often softening the curves in the spine by strengthening and lengthening the small muscles on the inside or outside of the curve. Nonstrenuous rotation exercises performed while sitting on the ball promote all the benefits of rotation while facilitating the actual act of sitting tall, which is difficult, even impossible, for many to do while sitting on a mat. The ball is unequaled in bringing the body back into balance before postural problems become neck, back, or hip problems that can be agonizing and costly.

What Is Ideal Posture?

What is ideal posture, or the optimal body alignment that we aspire to for health and attractiveness? First, cultivate an awareness of the three natural curves of the spine: the slightly concave curve of the cervical spine, or the neck; the slightly convex curve of the upper back; and the concave curve of the lower back.

These curves are essential: in conjunction with the gel-filled disks, they act as shock absorbers. When we retrain postural habits we are not trying to eliminate these natural curves. The goal is to avoid exaggerating them. We strive to maintain a neutral position of the pelvis where the front bones of the pelvis—the pubic bone and the front of the two hipbones—are in the same plane, again preserving the natural curve of the lumbar spine. The head, which weighs twelve to sixteen pounds, should balance squarely and with minimal effort on top of the spine. Remember: the skull extends into back space as well as front space.

Ideally there should be two opposing forces that work constantly through the body. When we ground the body while standing, or anchor the sitz bones while sitting, the upper body naturally lengthens and releases upward and outward. Even when we are lying on a mat these two opposing forces are at work. This feeling of opposition through the body is important for good body placement and posture.

Inside Out: The Postural Muscles

Strengthening the postural muscles—the small, deep muscles that run alongside the spine—will help support the larger muscles and bring the spine and body into balance. The superficial rectus abdominis and the long thoracolumbar extensors are similar to guy wires that balance the pole from the outside. Yet it is the deep muscles that provide the support in the links between each segment of the pole. If the small deep muscles do not work effectively to link each section of the pole, the flagpole will become unstable.

The principle of working from the inside out is essential to Pilates, and the ball is an excellent tool to help you implement this principle. Just sitting on the ball recruits deep muscles crucial to the stabilization of your joints and your spine. The stronger the small

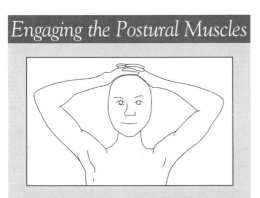

Engaging the Postural Muscles

*t*ry the following simple exercise. Lock your hands over your head. While extending the head upward gently resist the movement with your hands. This small movement helps activate the deep muscles, which are close to the vertebral column. These small, deep, postural muscles maintain an erect spine.

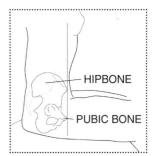

HIPBONE
PUBIC BONE

neutral spine

The goal of Pilates is not to try to flatten the back or create an exaggerated curve in the lower back, upper back, or neck. The goal is to preserve the natural curves of the spine without overtilting or tucking the pelvis. The neutral pelvis position, in which the pubic bone and the two hipbones are in the same plane, stabilizes the back so that the disks are in a safe position and are not compressed.

Place your hands on your pelvis or use a mirror as you do the pelvic-tilt exercise in "Sitting" (see page 33). Notice that you are moving the pelvis in and out of neutral.

31

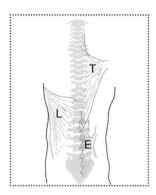

anatomy on the ball: spine muscles

The erector spinae are bands of muscles that run alongside your spine. These deep muscles are designed to work constantly to keep the spine erect. They take turns contracting so that their action is constant for sustained periods of time.

Latissimus dorsi is a large muscle that originates on the lower and midback, wraps around the trunk, and fastens onto the upper arm. Trapezius, another superficial back muscle, is a long diamond-shaped muscle of the neck and upper and midback. These large muscles are designed for powerful actions of brief duration.

deep muscles, the more forcefully the large superficial muscles, such as the "traps," the "lats," and the "glutes," will work while helping you kick, leap, and throw. If the deep muscle system does not supply inner support for outer muscles, the larger superficial muscles may be activated to take over the work of the small muscles. This can cause pain, among other problems, since these large muscles are not intended, for example, to hold the spine erect for prolonged periods of time.

Many of the exercises presented here contribute directly to postural improvements. Abdominal exercises (chapter 4) strengthen the core of the body; restorative exercises (chapter 7) stretch and strengthen the hip flexors, hamstrings, and muscles that run down the sides and backs of the legs; and the extension exercises (chapter 5) extend the space between each vertebra and strengthen the back muscles. In this chapter, however, I have chosen specific exercises and named them "postural" because they not only work the small postural muscles close to the spine, but they foster an awareness of spinal mobility through elongation, rotation, and sidebending.

The Postural Exercises

The following postural exercises are practiced while sitting on the ball. Sitting tall on the ball aligns the body naturally and safely and places the least strain on the body. The first exercise helps us to locate neutral pelvis; a mirror may be helpful in practicing this exercise, to make sure your pelvis is not tilted forward or backward. While performing Pelvic Tilts you will be moving the pelvis out of neutral. Sometimes moving the pelvis forward or backward out of neutral helps many students to locate neutral pelvis.

Take care with rib cage placement with these exercises. Is the rib cage full and unrestricted, to permit proper breathing? Try not to allow the rib cage to lift upward or collapse downward. One final point: ideal posture, whether lying on a mat or sitting on the ball, is assisted by the abdominal connection. We are not just activating the superficial rectus abdominis, but the deep transversus abdominus as well. (More on the abdominals follows in the next chapter.)

Sitting

Sitting on a ball is active work, and therefore better for your posture and general back health than collapsing into a chair. When sitting on the ball, hips and knees should be bent at 90-degree angles. Do not let your feet get too close to the ball. Feet should be just wider than hip-distance apart to create a strong base of support. Yes, you can slump on the ball, but you will be aware of it because slumping increases the ball's instability.

Purpose To find optimal posture. To learn mobility through the spine and to become familiar with neutral pelvis.

Watchpoints • In ordinary sitting (movement 1), avoid overarching the back and popping out the rib cage. • Unassisted sitting is an endurance activity, so do not overdo it. • Keep the chin horizontal, eyes level. • Do not force movement 2. Stop if there is any pain.

reach through the tops of the ears

We want a long neck but not a forced or strained neck. When you read "lengthen through the tops of the ears," think of opening disks in the cervical spine (the neck) but keeping the chin horizontal at the same time. Imagine you are in a theater and attempting to read the subtitles above a tall person in front of you. Eye gaze is straight ahead.

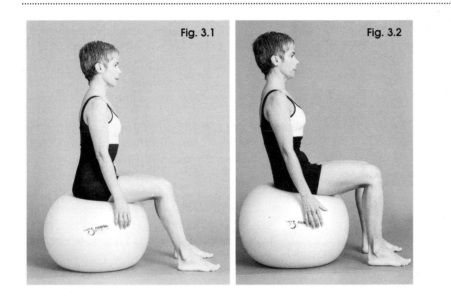

Fig. 3.1   Fig. 3.2

starting position

Sit on the center of your ball, knees aligned with ankles, legs just wider than hip-distance apart and parallel. Feet are firmly planted, toes long and relaxed. Chin is level (fig. 3.1). Think of pulling the navel up and into the back of the spine.

movement 1: sitting

1. Relax the shoulders.
2. As fingertips relax toward the floor, let the weight of the body drop into the ball.
3. Lengthen through the tops of the ears (see sidebar).

4. Check your posture in a mirror or with your fingers. Notice if the three natural curves of the spine are in place, or whether you are flattening or exaggerating any of them.
5. Sit for a number of minutes, breathing slowly and deeply. Add time as you get stronger.

movement 2: pelvic tilt

1. Sit on the center of your ball, knees aligned with ankles, legs just wider than hip-distance apart and parallel. Feet are firmly planted, toes long and relaxed. Chin is level.

2. Keeping your feet firmly planted, curl the tailbone forward and let the ball roll slightly forward under you (fig. 3.2). Return to neutral pelvis.
3. Push your tailbone back and roll the ball backward.
4. Repeat this movement four to six times. Notice how you are moving the pelvis in and out of neutral.

Bouncing

A bounce can be added to the sitting position. Place a chair nearby to steady yourself if you are afraid of losing your balance. Bounce as vigorously as is comfortable. Bouncing aligns the spine in its most efficient position and improves the endurance of the postural muscles. Never bend, twist, or rotate the spine while bouncing. Jumping jacks, shoulder shrugs, and many arm and leg movements seen in an aerobics class can be transferred to your ball. See chapter 9 for ideas for a low-impact cardiovascular workout.

Purpose To train and improve the endurance of postural muscles.
Watchpoints • Never combine rotation or bending of the spine with bouncing.
• You should always be able to carry on a conversation. If not, slow the bounce.

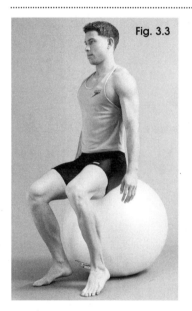

Fig. 3.3

starting position

Sit on the center of your ball, knees aligned with ankles, legs just wider than hip-distance apart and parallel. Feet are firmly planted, toes long and relaxed. Chin is level. Think of pulling the navel up and into the back of the spine.

movement

1. Press your feet to the floor, activate the thigh muscles, and bounce as vigorously as is comfortable (fig. 3.3). Relax and breathe as you bounce.
2. When you stop bouncing, sit tall and check your feet and ankles. Use a mirror or your fingers to be sure that you are in neutral spine. There is a curve in the lower back but not an exaggerated curve. The neck is long but not tense. The ears are aligned over the shoulders.

Where Are My Sitz Bones?

*t*he sitz bones are the bones you sit on. To find the sitz bones, or ischial tuberosities, sit on your ball or the ground, place your hand under one buttock, and move the fleshly part to one side. Palpate the little rocker on the bottom of that pelvic half. The sitz bones are not a part of the thigh, as some think. Your weight should be distributed evenly on these rockers. These are your feet when you are not on your feet!

Now that you have found optimal posture here are some more exercises to help you maintain it.

Spine Stretch Forward

This is a highly controlled release of the spine with maximum abdominal connection: we are not collapsing. The head moves first—it slowly rolls away from the top joint. Then you sequence through the rest of the spine. Spine Stretch Forward is also a breathing exercise. Allow all the air to leave the lungs on the exhale. Breathe back into the rib cage on the inhale. Try not to let the ball roll.

Purpose To stretch the spine. To coordinate breath with movement.
Watchpoints • Keep navel-to-spine connection throughout the move.
• Maintain a C curve at the bottom; don't collapse down. • Keep the chin from digging into the chest.

*In coming up
and going down,
roll your spine like a wheel.
Vertebra by vertebra,
try to roll and unroll.
—Joseph H. Pilates*

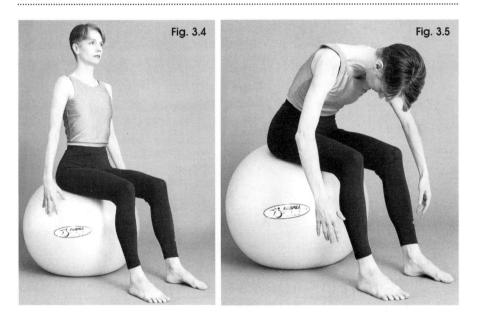

Fig. 3.4   Fig. 3.5

starting position

Sit erect on your ball (neutral pelvis) (fig. 3.4). Think of pulling your belly button up and into the back of the spine.

movement

1. Inhale to lengthen through the tops of the ears.
2. Exhale to drop the chin, sink the sternum back, and roll down one vertebra at a time (fig. 3.5).
3. Inhale at the bottom to fill the back rib cage.
4. Exhale to curl back up, stacking the vertebrae; the head will float on top like a balloon.
5. Do five Spine Stretches, connecting movement with breath.

35

The Saw

This is a wonderful postural exercise that utilizes rotation to activate the small postural muscles of the spine. When the Saw is done on a ball it's even more effective, because if you slouch or relax your abdominals the ball will drift.

Purpose To restore and maintain good posture.

Watchpoints • Hipbones should remain centered on the ball. • Keep both sitz bones firmly anchored on the ball. • Don't let your arms drift behind your torso. • Keep both shoulders down.

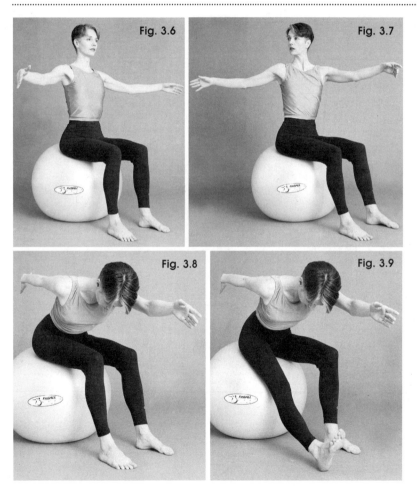

Fig. 3.6 Fig. 3.7

Fig. 3.8 Fig. 3.9

starting position

1. Sit erect on your sitz bones. Position your legs just wider than hip-distance apart, feet parallel and in line with the knees.
2. Open your arms to the sides (fig. 3.6).

movement 1: the saw

1. Inhale and rotate to the right as you get taller (fig. 3.7).
2. Exhale and stretch your left arm diagonally over your right leg, aiming your left hand about two feet above and in line with your right baby toe. Let your head follow your arm. The head should stay aligned on the spine (fig. 3.8).
3. Inhale and slowly roll up one vertebra at a time to a rotated position (fig. 3.7).
4. Exhale as you rotate very tall back to the center (fig. 3.6).
5. Repeat three times on each side.

movement 2: the saw with hamstring stretch

1. Inhale and rotate to the right (fig. 3.7) as you get taller.
2. Exhale and straighten the leg, pressing the heel into the floor and lifting the toes as you stretch diagonally over your right baby toe (fig. 3.9). You will feel the hamstrings stretch.
3. Inhale to slowly roll up to a rotated position. Plant the foot back into place.
4. Exhale as you rotate very tall back to the center (fig. 3.6).
5. Repeat three times on each side.

Round Back

Here we are using abdominal strength to stabilize and roll through the spine. Remember you are not rolling back very far. Simply roll slightly back off your sitz bones, maintaining a strong C curve of the abdominals. The ball rolls a little forward with this exercise.

Purpose To roll through the back keeping the abdominals connected.

Watchpoints • Be sure that you roll through the spine and do not hyperextend or arch through the lower back. • Keep shoulders sliding down the back.

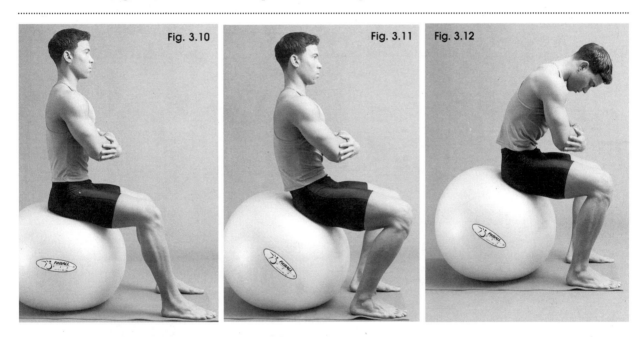

Fig. 3.10   Fig. 3.11   Fig. 3.12

starting position

1. Sit tall on your sitz bones on the center of the ball (neutral pelvis), feet just wider than hip-distance apart and firmly planted.
2. Grasp your elbows, positioning arms just below the rib cage (fig. 3.10).

movement

1. Inhale to lengthen through the tops of the ears.
2. Exhale to roll the sitz bones slightly under you. Inhale and stay (fig. 3.11).
3. Exhale to increase the curve in the abdominals as you roll the top of the body over the legs (fig. 3.12).
4. Inhale to roll up to a tall sitting position (neutral pelvis).
5. Repeat four times.

BodySpheres—Seated Lateral Shift

*m*ari Naumovski has been exploring movement with balls since 1988 when she first discovered them during the course of her movement training in New York City. The Seated Lateral Shift is initiated in the pelvic area, specifically from the sitz bones. Move slowly, especially as you rotate to guide the ball beneath you. Mari says that this exercise shows how the pelvic area is the weight center around which the rest of the body organizes to support a well-executed movement.

Sit tall on your sitz bones on the center of the ball (neutral pelvis). Inhale to prepare. Exhale to shift your pelvis directly to the right (fig. 3.13). Inhale to shift to the center. Exhale to shift the pelvis directly to the left.

Now we go further: this time shift the pelvis farther to the right until your pelvis rolls on to your left outer hip. Your feet will swivel and your whole body will now roll to the left. To catch yourself from rolling off the ball place both hands on the ball, just outside your left thigh (fig. 3.14). Inhale and stay, then exhale to shift your hips directly sideways to the left to return your whole body to the center. Repeat on the opposite side.

Mari Naumovski notes: Notice that you can only move sideways so far until your pelvis rotates in the opposite direction, causing your body as a whole to respond to this spiral orientation.

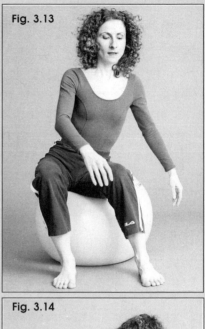

Fig. 3.13

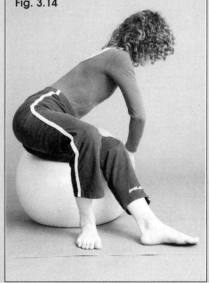

Fig. 3.14

Spine Twist

This twist is done in a tall position. Try and keep the hips directly centered on the ball during the rotation; if your knees have moved so have your hips, and you have gone too far in rotation. Start with your arms crossed and low to keep the shoulders down and to be sure that the rotation is happening in the spine, not in the arms or head. Think tall, taller, tallest!

Purpose To rotate while trying to keep length through the spine.
Watchpoints • Keep the rotation very small if you have any lower back pain. • Notice whether your degree of rotation is the same on both sides.

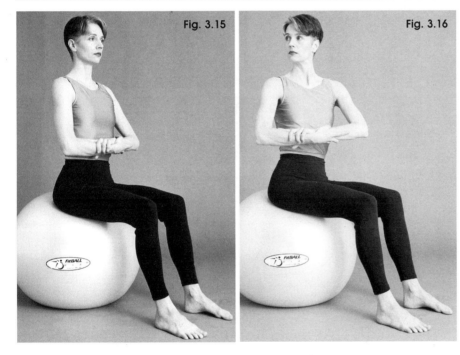

Fig. 3.15   Fig. 3.16

rotation: nutrition for your disks

Let your spine come alive and be energized with gentle twists! When you rotate the body in a horizontal plane the vertebral disks naturally compress, which means there is a reduction in the overall height of the disk. Some areas of the spine are built more for rotation than other sections, so it is important to keep rotations controlled and to think about elongating through the spine rather than twisting the spine. If you have lower back pain or disk problems rotate with caution.

starting position

Sit on your sitz bones on the center of the ball (neutral pelvis), feet parallel and just wider than hip-distance apart. Arms are crossed and low (fig. 3.15).

movement 1

1. Inhale to prepare.
2. Exhale to rotate as you get taller (fig. 3.16).
3. Inhale to return to the center.
4. Repeat on the other side.
Do three sets.

movement 2

1. Open your arms, palms down, and repeat movement 1.
2. Do three sets.

Mermaid

Sidebending is a necessary part of any workout. Think more of elongation than bending. Do this stretch slowly and cautiously so that you maintain height through the spine and do not roll off the ball.

Purpose To bend the spine laterally.
Watchpoints • Do not arch the back; keep the hips and ribs in one line. Elongate the spine; do not simply bend or crunch sideways. • Keep the head in line with the spine.

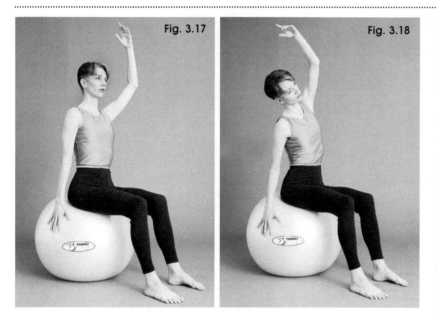

Fig. 3.17   Fig. 3.18

starting position
Sit tall on the center of your ball (neutral pelvis), one hand on the side of the ball, the other out to the side.

movement
1. Inhale to float the left arm up; the left shoulder remains down (fig. 3.17).
2. Exhale to elongate to the right (fig. 3.18).
3. Inhale to return to the center by reaching through the tops of the ears.
4. Exhale as the left arm drops down.
5. Inhale to lift the right arm up; the right shoulder slides down the back.
6. Exhale to elongate to the left.
7. Inhale to return to the center.
8. Repeat three times on each side.

Did you notice if bending to one side felt easier than the other side? The key to good posture is overall body fitness and awareness. In the next chapter the Pilates on the Ball abdominal exercises will complement the postural exercises by providing crucial support for the spine. The abdominal exercises are specially designed to firm the abdomen and build a strong core. A strong core not only maintains good posture, but it helps heal and prevent lower back pain and problems.

4

The Abdominal Exercises

The body is a sacred garment. It's your first and last garment; it is what you enter life in and what you depart life with, and it should be treated with honor.
—Martha Graham

Edwin's Story

Edwin was a student activist in the highly charged political climate of 1980s South African politics. When he was in his mid-twenties and on the run from an apartheid army that wanted to recruit him forcibly to fight for a regime he despised, he noticed that he was beginning to wake up to lower back pain each morning. Some days he found it hard to get out of bed. Often, after a long car ride or sitting too long at a meeting, his back suddenly seized up. Doctors gave him a physical, even ordered X rays, but nothing showed up. A coworker, also an activist, was studying massage therapy and offered to examine him. She noted that the muscles that ran vertically down either side of his spine were hard and in a state of contraction. He kept insisting that he had a "weak back," but this therapist trainee disagreed. Edwin, she explained, had strong tense muscles that were tired and overworked. He needed to relax and let his muscles go. What he really needed was to flee from the intense mental and physical tension of living in a country where he could be arrested for carrying a Nelson Mandela T-shirt in the trunk of his car.

More than a decade later the walls of apartheid had come down, and South Africa had gone through a miraculous transformation. Edwin was settled in an African National Congress–related job and a loving relationship. The country had opened up and new ideas, including health-related practices, were flowing in. Edwin visited an acupuncturist, trained in Japan and New York, who inserted needles in appropriate meridians whenever his back acted up. Unfortunately his back still acted up—a lot. The extraordinary strains of his youth had now changed to the typical stresses of any North American life—waiting too long in checkout lines; fighting rush-hour traffic; coping with work deadlines and office politics, which Edwin joked were political tensions with a little *p*. But he now had the money to book some treatment time with a registered massage therapist; she made the same observation that the trainee had made twelve years earlier—that the muscles in his lower back were chronically contracted. In addition, Edwin now suffered stomachaches and insomnia.

When Edwin and I worked together we started with tailbone and pelvis placement. I showed him how to find neutral pelvis and explained how neutral pelvis stabilizes the lower back so that the disks are in a safe position and are not compressed. For Edwin, like many people, finding neutral pelvis meant lessening the curve in his lower back. Then he showed me the sit-ups he had been doing for years at his local gym. He had been doing many repetitions with rapid speed. Typical sit-ups and abdominal machines strengthen the superficial rectus abdominis muscle, a muscle not designed for supporting the back. In addition, in full sit-ups the powerful hip flexors aid the movement.

Vigorous movements without the proper activation of deep abdominal muscles can aggravate lower back pain. I taught Edwin how to make the sit-ups much smaller (and slower) and how to ensure that the pelvis is kept in neutral. Neutral pelvis helps facilitate the deeper contraction of the circular, waist-narrowing transversus abdominis, the deepest of the four abdominal muscles.

Edwin and I also worked on back breathing. Like many students, he wanted to know why the breath is going into the rib cage and not the abdominals. I reminded him that if the breath were flowing into the belly it would release the belly. We want the opposite: connected abdominals that wrap themselves tightly around the middle and protect the lower back.

I also encouraged Edwin to find ways to eliminate stress and to slow down, breathe, and stretch. He did his Pilates on the Ball abdominal exercises every day. He also began to write about his experiences of growing up in apartheid South Africa. Soreness eventually began to disappear. Head- and stomachaches were less frequent as he committed to taking time to enjoy life instead of focusing on the chaos and excitement of his new world. "My back feels better than it ever did," he wrote to me a few months later.

Life and Lower Back Pain

Of all the students I see each week, lower back pain, dull or severe, is the single most frequently heard complaint. Elite and recreational athletes, actors, housewives, students, and professionals all suffer from a wide array of lower back syndromes and strains. Less frequently back pain can be a result of structural abnormalities, but it more commonly involves postural muscles, tendons, ligaments, or nerves. For many people lower back pain is chronic and debilitating.

Often the pain is related to tension, stress, and psychological factors. By the time I worked with Edwin he admitted he had a strong fear of recurrent back-pain attacks. This fear in itself can aggravate pain. Many people have a relationship of fear with pain. Even after the pain vacates their bodies they curtail activities for fear of bringing on another attack.

There are many causes of lower back pain—many more than can be explored within the scope of this book. When the pain is a direct result of an injury, accident, or fall—a real-life calamity that the sufferer can identify—the chances of recovery are better. There is a satisfaction in being able to account for the pain, and most people in this category are inclined to take the necessary steps to regain their health and mobility. The very real trauma of a car accident forces them to act: they have been wronged by others or by their own misjudgment or carelessness and now have no choice but to fix and restore their bodies.

Unfortunately the majority of people who suffer from lower back pain may not be able to account for their misery. Dragging a brush through their hair

Neutral Pelvis and Back-Pain Relief

*t*his time we are trying to find neutral pelvis while lying on a mat. Lie on your back, knees bent, feet in line with the knees, knees in line with the hips. Make sure the pubic bone and the two hipbones on the front of the pelvis are flat and in the same plane. The goal is to encourage the spine to rest into its natural curves and, if necessary, to lessen the curve in the lower back. Feel the tailbone as heavy and lengthening without forcing it down on the mat.

Try slipping a hand under your lower back. With most body shapes you should be able to ease your fingers into the space between the floor and your back. ("Ease" being the operative word here—it is desirable that this space be smaller rather than gaping.)

Add a ball to this exercise to soothe you when you have lower back pain. Slip a ball under your knees. Allow the back to settle with gravity, not force. Try to maintain the pose at least twenty minutes, even longer if possible. Practice rib cage or abdominal breathing. Focus on the internal sensations: Is one side of the pelvis more settled than the other?

Come out of this position carefully. Roll on to your side, pull your knees to your chest, and slowly use your hands to bring you to sitting.

can trigger the same amount of pain as falling on ice. "Life" or "aging" are sometimes the explanations given, often taken from the lips of doctors. "I'm not getting any younger," they claim with a sigh, as if there is nothing in their power to help them rediscover their full potential as human beings. In all fairness, as any doctor or health care practitioner can attest, the body *is* a mystery and it may be undermined by a multitude of unexplained symptoms that do not respond to medical treatments. Undiagnosable pain is frustrating and settles over every aspect of the sufferer's life. In fact, when these people sigh that "life" is the cause of their stiff ankles, tension headaches, and lower back pain they are correct. There are continual, unabated tensions and traumas in our environment, and if these powerful stresses are allowed to continue they will eventually cause disease and physical complications.

The Powerhouse and Lower Back Pain

The good news is that by changing behavior and strengthening the abdominals, especially the deep, stabilizing abdominal muscles as well as the more superficial ones, lower back pain can be avoided. Yet most daily activities—even the most popular sports—do not strengthen this area.

Joseph Pilates saw the abdominal area, the area between the bottom rib and the pelvis, as the center, or powerhouse, of the body. He perceived this "girdle of strength" as a physical, gravitational center as well as a spiritual or mental one. One of the fundamental principles behind the acclaimed Pilates Method of conditioning is that the powerhouse is the center of all movement. The stronger the powerhouse, the more powerful and efficient the movement. Moreover, when the abdominal muscles are strong they keep the spine properly aligned and support and distribute the stresses placed on it.

There are three abdominal muscles that work with the small spinal muscles of the erector spinae group to make up the powerhouse. The superficial rectus abdominis muscle is responsible for flexing the trunk by pulling the ribs toward the pelvis; it has, with the other abdominals, a postural role. The deeper transversus abdominis is a muscle group that stabilizes the lumbar spine by narrowing the abdominal wall and is associated with the prevention of chronic lower back pain. If you place your hands around your waist and cough you will feel the transversus tighten. The external and internal obliques, often referred to as the body's natural corset because of the way these sheetlike muscles crisscross the body, are responsible for sidebending and twisting of the spine. A weakness in any of these abdominal muscles will have an effect on the stability of the lower back and can cause pain in that area.

Centering

Pilates on the Ball and other mind/body holistic exercise systems can help people relearn how to engage and utilize abdominals and control hypertense muscles. However, it is not enough to exercise our bodies. We need to exercise our minds against the battering and accumulative effects of trauma and stress. Joseph Pilates knew this. When he designed his highly effective method of mental and physical conditioning, he fused the best from Eastern and Western philosophies of exercise, aiming for a perfect harmony of body, mind, and spirit.

Pilates believed that all movement had to be initiated from the powerhouse, or center. The stronger the powerhouse, the more effective the movement. This process is called centering, and it is an essential principle in Pilates on the Ball. Centering is also referred to as "navel-to-spine." How I wish I had known about centering, or navel-to-spine, all those years ago when I studied ballet. If I had initiated from the powerhouse and drawn my belly button up and into my spine, how much stronger and more secure my pirouettes would have been. I was never taught how to create a firm and strong abdomen or how to find my center, so I spun around like Earth on its axis. Even a washing machine rattles and shakes dangerously when it is off balance.

Centering on the mat, or on the ball, cannot help but transfer a clarity and tranquillity that will help in all sorts of life situations. In a world of constant stimuli and chaos we can easily lose focus and become unhinged. Pilates on the Ball helps us to become centered and at peace. Whatever one's definition of being centered is, the physical cannot help but inspire the spirit, making us more capable of accepting change and challenge. What can be more awesome than draping your fifty-something-year-old body over an oversized beach ball for the first time in forty years?

Centering is crucial when we climb on the ball. In fact it may be one of the most fundamental ingredients for effective and safe ballwork! Without working effectively from the powerhouse, how will we balance and maneuver on this mobile piece of equipment? If we are not centered, if our abdominals are not engaged, the ball will drift easily. Moreover, if we initiate from other parts of the body and not from the powerhouse, we can injure ourselves or be unable to accomplish the movement effectively.

The Abdominal Exercises

Pilates on the Ball is great therapy for lower back pain. Most of the following exercises can be done even if you experience modest lower back pain, but take care to stay with the modifications. The abdominal exercises are your warm-up

The Pilates Method is a flowing motion outward from a strong center.
—Romana Kryzanowska, premiere Pilates trainer, The Pilates Studio, New York

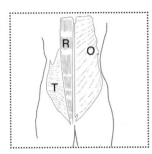

anatomy on the ball: abdominal muscles

Transversus abdominis is the deepest of the four abdominal muscles. It wraps horizontally around your waist and stabilizes the lumbar spine by narrowing the abdominal wall. This muscle has attracted a lot of attention lately because of its association with the prevention of lower back pain. The long, superficial rectus abdominis runs up from the pubic bone to the bottom of the sternum and lower rib cartilages. It is responsible for flexing the trunk; it's not really functional in supporting the back. The external and internal obliques, the natural corset of the body, are responsible for sidebending and twisting the spine.

The abdominal muscles—especially the transversus—and the deep spinal muscles make up the Pilates powerhouse or "girdle of strength." When the abdominal core is strong we prevent lower back pain and can safely and efficiently perform movements of the arms and legs.

exercises: they strengthen the abdominals as well as prepare you for the more strenuous movements to come. Remember to use your breath, especially the exhale, to help engage the abdominals. If you have neck tension, keep the head down on the mat where I indicate to do so and avoid using the ball, since its one and a half to two pounds of resistance may aggravate the neck. Yet the stronger the abdominals become the less tension you will experience in the neck. Also take care to stabilize the shoulders, easing them down and back, before you do any movement, especially before lifting or rolling the ball. You will notice in Pilates on the Ball that we only do six to eight repetitions of each exercise. Joseph Pilates was quite adamant about the number of reps. He called overworking the muscles an "infraction" that creates muscular burnout, fatigue, and "poison" in the muscles. It is the quality of the movement that is important, not the quantity.

Navel-to-Spine

The four-point kneeling position is an effective position in which to teach the action of drawing the lower abdominals up and in. When I speak of navel-to-spine I tell my students to imagine a thick cord connecting the belly button to the back of the spine. Other teachers use the image of a tiny ice pick poking into the lower belly to get their students to hollow out the abdominals. First we practice lifting the belly button up and then releasing it onto the ball. Then we learn to keep the navel-to-spine connection for both the inhale and exhale as we add simple arm movements.

Purpose To learn how to create a strong center by finding and engaging the abdominals.

Watchpoints • This movement is subtle. The contraction of the abdominals is performed in a slow, controlled manner. The buttock muscles are not involved. • Avoid arching the back or moving the pelvis. Keep the hips on the ball; eye gaze is at the floor. • Keep shoulders easing down the back.
• Remember to inhale through the nose, exhale through the mouth.

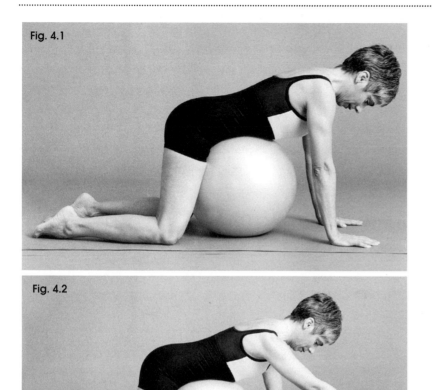

Fig. 4.1

Fig. 4.2

what's wrong with traditional sit-ups?

Typical sit-ups and abdominal machines strengthen the superficial rectus abdominis muscle, a muscle that is not crucial for supporting the back. In addition, in full sit-ups the powerful hip flexors aid the movement, so you get strong hip flexors instead of strong deep abdominal muscles as desired. Many repetitions with rapid speed can aggravate lower back pain. Crunches can also pull the neck and round the shoulders, causing neck pain.

starting position

Lie over your ball. Be sure that your weight is equally distributed on all four limbs; hands are directly beneath the shoulders, knees beneath the hips (fig. 4.1). If you have a large ball you may have your weight on your toes rather than your knees. Keep your head aligned on the spine—the eye gaze will be down.

movement 1

1. Inhale to lengthen through the spine.
2. Exhale to lift your navel.
3. Inhale to release and drop your navel onto the ball.
4. Exhale to lift the navel.
5. Inhale to the drop navel.
6. Repeat this movement five times.

movement 2: with hand lifts

1. Inhale to lengthen through the spine.

2. Exhale to lift your navel.
3. Inhale to lift one hand a few inches off the ground (fig. 4.2). Keep the abdominals connected.
4. Exhale to lower the arm.
5. Inhale to lift the second hand.
6. Exhale to lower.
7. Repeat four times on each side, keeping the abdominals connected for both in and out breaths.

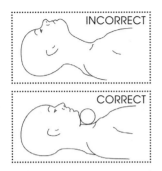

**head position
on the mat**

When lying on your back
be sure your head is not
tilted so far that your neck
arches. You may need to
drop the chin gently for-
ward as if you have a tennis ball held at the throat.
This correction will pro-
duce a sensation of
lengthening through the
neck, which is what we
want when the head is on
the mat. This is what I
mean by the directive
"lengthen through the
back of the neck." In
some cases a flat pillow
may be necessary.

To lift the head safely,
first nod or drop the chin
forward and curve your
head up immediately as
you empty the air from
the lungs. Avoid sticking
your chin into the air or
grinding it into the chest,
for that puts a lot of pressure on the back of the
neck. Make sure your
gaze is on your thighs and
not on the ceiling when
the head is up.

48

Little Abdominal Curls

This is the first in a series of highly effective abdominal exercises. This exercise will teach you how to curl the upper body while keeping the navel-to-
spine connection. This small exercise is so much more efficient than hooking
your feet under a couch and heaving yourself through a series of sit-ups, which
creates strong hip flexors, not abdominals. Hands placed behind the head will
help you to practice safely lifting the head from the mat. Try to keep your
pelvis in neutral and not tuck up the tailbone. If you have never done Pilates
before, you may find the moves to be much slower than you are used to.

Purpose To strengthen the abdominal muscles. To learn to lift the head off
the mat. To help ease mild lower back pain.

Watchpoints • Try to use the abdominals, not the hands, to lift the head.
• Try not to let the chin dig into the chest. • Keep the pelvis in neutral.

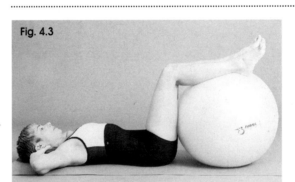

Fig. 4.3

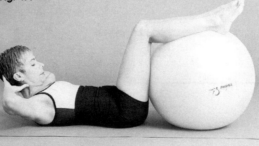

Fig. 4.4

starting position

1. Lie on your back with the
ball under your knees, knees
in line with your hips.
2. Check that the back of
the neck is in "lengthened
position." Place hands
behind the head, elbows
wide (fig. 4.3).

movement

1. Inhale to prepare and
begin to drop the chin while
the head is still on the mat.
2. Exhale to lift the head,
flexing the upper body.
3. Inhale and stay; your gaze
is at your thighs, not at the
ceiling (fig 4.4).
4. Exhale to return your head
to the mat.
5. Repeat eight times, slow
and controlled.

Full Abdominal Curls

The transition from the previous exercise into full abdominal curls is to pick the ball up with your feet and lift it into the air, passing the ball to your hands. If this is not possible simply roll the ball beside you and then pick it up with your hands. Eventually you will master the essential Pilates principle of flow, but right now it is enough to remember that ideally one movement should flow into the next one. The more you go through the exercises, the easier it will be for you to master the flow. At this stage, don't worry about perfection; just try the movements.

Purpose To strengthen the abdominal muscles. To learn to lift the head safely from the mat without using the hands. To help ease mild lower back pain.

Watchpoints • Be sure that the chin nods and then the head comes up immediately, chin to chest, without grinding into the chest. • Be sure that the abdominals are working. Press them with your fingers to see that they are engaged. • Do not flex too high, as you'll engage the powerful hip flexors. • Keep the pelvis in neutral. Do not let the tailbone lift off the mat. • Relax, in good alignment, between each exercise.

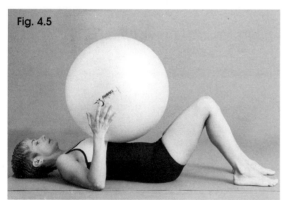

Fig. 4.5

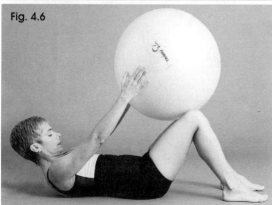

Fig. 4.6

starting position

1. Lie on your back with your knees bent and feet on the floor, sitz-bone distance apart.
2. Place the ball on your rib cage and hold it with both hands (fig. 4.5).
3. Sense that the back of the neck is lengthening.

movement

1. Inhale to prepare and begin to nod the chin.
2. Exhale to lift the head and flex the upper body, rolling the ball up your thighs.
3. Inhale and stay; your gaze is on the thigh, not the ceiling (fig. 4.6).
4. Exhale to roll back, head to mat.
5. Repeat eight times, slow and controlled.

49

BodySpheres—Upper Abdominal Curl against the Wall

Sit on your ball facing a wall. Your toes should be about one and a half the length of your foot away from the wall. Tilt your pelvis backward so your torso curls and place one foot on the wall directly in front of your hip. Repeat with the other foot. Keep your hands on the ball for extra support.

Walk your feet up the wall until your legs are stretched. As you inhale, place your hands behind your head and lengthen your upper back (fig. 4.7). Exhale to curl your upper body (fig. 4.8). Take care to leave space between your chin and chest to avoid pressing your head down with the force of your arms. Don't let your head drop when you extend your head back.

Repeat four to six times. Mari Naumovski notes: This exercise takes advantage of the eccentric part of the muscle contraction. In eccentric contraction, the muscle is lengthening out of its shortened position. It requires tremendous strength to control this movement smoothly. You are also getting a deep hamstring stretch as your legs are "sandwiched" between the wall and your torso.

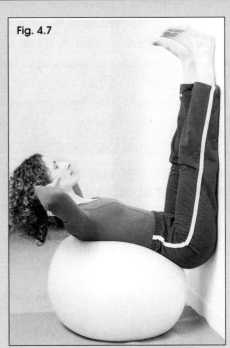
Fig. 4.7

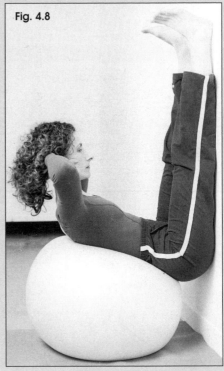
Fig. 4.8

The Waterfall

If you have no lower back pain we will take the Full Abdominal Curls one step further and roll the ball up and over the knees to the ankles. Keep your shoulders stabilized when you roll the ball along the trunk or the legs: don't let having the hands on the ball cause the shoulders to lift to the ears. The shape of the ball helps us embody the wheel image that is used in so many of the Pilates exercises. Try not to simply go through the motions—feel the spine rolling and unrolling; feel one bone at a time as it contacts the mat. The ball helps us slow down and feel the movement inside and outside the body.

Purpose To strengthen the abdominal muscles. To experience the spine unrolling like a wheel.

Watchpoints • If the feet are too close to your buttocks they will hamper you from getting the ball up and over the knees. • Keep the ball in contact with the body and feel the sensation of the ball on the body. • If you have lower back pain do not let the ball go past the knees; keep the knees bent. • Keep the abdomen flat and hollowed; remember: navel-to-spine. • Keep the shoulders down and back.

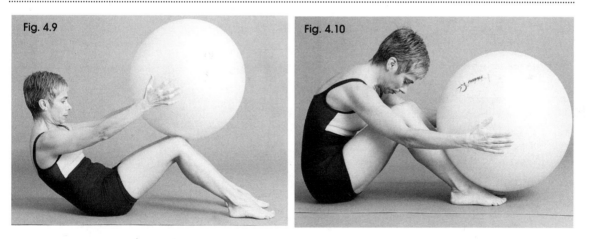

Fig. 4.9   Fig. 4.10

starting position

1. Lie on your back with knees bent and feet on the floor, sitz-bone distance apart.
2. Place your ball on the rib cage and hold it with both hands. Be sure that the feet are not too close to the buttocks.

movement

1. Inhale to lengthen on the mat.
2. Exhale to lift the head and flex the upper body as you roll the ball up the thighs (fig. 4.9), over the knees, and down the shins (fig. 4.10).
3. Inhale when the ball is at the ankles as you begin to roll back.

4. Exhale to continue releasing back, rolling the ball over the body, eventually releasing the head to the mat.
5. Repeat six times, slow and controlled.

The Rollup

Try to keep the ball off the body throughout this exercise, unlike with the Waterfall. Keeping the ball in the air will add resistance and make your abdominals work very hard. The ball also heightens your awareness of where your body is in space and adds an element of grace and fun to the exercise. Do not let the ball distract you from rolling your spine like a wheel and the other fundamentals of this exercise. Imagine that the abdominals are brakes slowing the unrolling of the spine. Keep the knees bent if you have lower back pain and avoid movement 2, the Full Rollup.

Purpose To strengthen the abdominals and learn to keep these muscles flat. To experience a hamstring and spine stretch in movement 2.

Watchpoints • Be sure that the shoulders slide down the back and that you do not arch the back off the mat when you take the ball overhead. • Sink the belly button into the spine to roll down one bone at a time. • Flex the feet in movement 2 and push the heels away from the hips for a hamstring stretch.

starting position

1. If you have lower back pain, keep your knees bent during this exercise. Lie flat on your back, legs together, holding the ball between your hands (fig. 4.11).

2. Keeping your shoulder blades on the mat, take the ball overhead (fig. 4.12). If the knees are bent be sure that the heels are not too close to your buttocks.

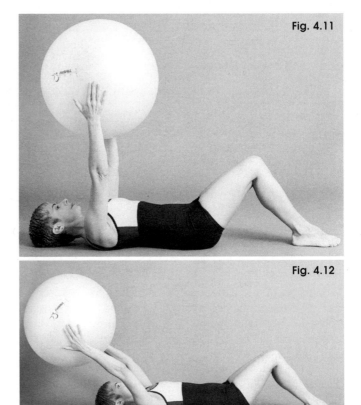

Fig. 4.11

Fig. 4.12

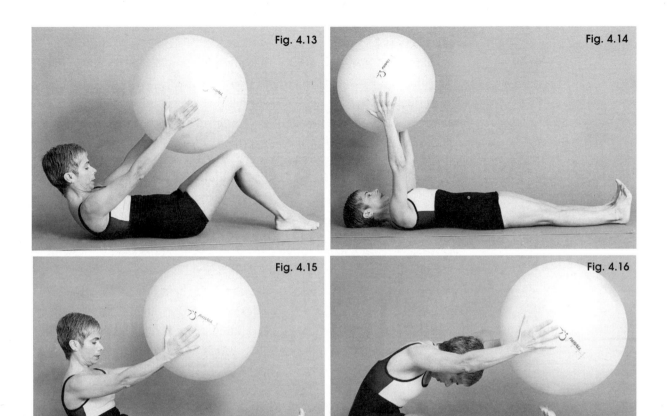

Fig. 4.13   Fig. 4.14

Fig. 4.15   Fig. 4.16

movement 1: half rollup

1. Inhale to lift the ball to the ceiling, head still on the mat.
2. Exhale to flex the body up, chin to chest, bringing the ball just above the knees (fig. 4.13).
3. Inhale to start to lift the ball back.
4. Exhale to roll back down one bone at a time.
5. Repeat six to eight times.

movement 2: full rollup

1. Inhale to lift the ball to the ceiling (fig. 4.14).
2. Exhale to flex the body up, peeling away from the mat one vertebra at a time (fig. 4.15).
3. Inhale to extend the ball toward your toes, and start to roll back pulling your navel toward your spine (fig. 4.16).
4. Exhale to reverse the movement, rolling down one vertebra at a time.
5. When your shoulder blades reach the mat, the ball floats back overhead.
6. Repeat six to eight times.

Leg Circles

The following is a subtle exercise that gives life and health to the ball-and-socket joint in the hip and can be done even with modest lower back pain. Start off with small circles, the leg in the air slightly bent. Think of drawing the circle with the knee, not the foot. Imagine you are drawing the face of a clock with your knee, making sure to cross through three o'clock, six o'clock, nine o'clock, and twelve o'clock. As you become more proficient the leg will get straighter, the circles will become larger, and you will think of the foot drawing the circle, not the knee. Because your other leg is resting on the ball you will be able to feel any wobbling in the pelvis. Remember: we want a calm, neutral pelvis.

Purpose To keep the femur moving freely in its ball-and-socket joint while the pelvis remains absolutely anchored.

Watchpoints • Keep the circles small and the leg bent at first. Eventually the leg will get straighter and the circles larger. • Use navel-to-spine to keep the pelvis calm and anchored. • Leg, or knee, crosses inward, across the body, the same distance as it crosses outward. • The leg on the ball should remain parallel and not turn in or out. • Shoulders should be relaxed and sliding down the back.

Modification If you have trouble keeping your leg in the air or feeling the shape of the circle, use a towel around the back of the thigh to guide the motion. Remember the correct placement of the head on the mat. You may need to gently drop the chin as if you are holding a tennis ball on the throat.

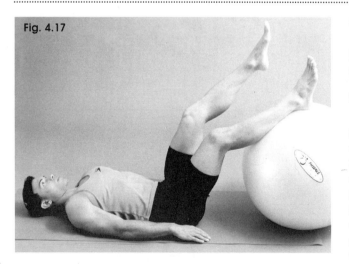

Fig. 4.17

starting position

1. Lie on your back, knees bent and on the ball, legs sitz-bone distance apart.
2. Slide the shoulders down. Place hands by your side.

movement

1. Inhale to prepare.
2. Exhale to lift the right knee off the ball so that it is directly above your hips (fig. 4.17).
3. Inhale to cross the knee inward, across the body.
4. Exhale to cross the knee outward and around to starting position.
5. Do five circles clockwise, inhaling for half the circle, exhaling for the other half of the circle.
6. Do five circles counterclockwise and repeat on the opposite leg. Don't be afraid to let the moving leg brush against the ball.

Rolling Like a Ball

From the Leg Circles starting position, pick the ball up between the feet and transport it to your hands. If you are able, do a Full Rollup to come up in place for Rolling Like a Ball, or roll on your side and use your hands to help you come into place. Rolling Like a Ball is a massage of the spine. Movement 2 teaches you to roll back off your sitz bones and hold yourself from rolling all the way back by using your abdominals. If you have no lower back pain do this version, practicing first without the ball. The ball helps you keep your heels close to your buttocks to maintain the correct tight "ball" position, but it is considerably more difficult with the ball than without.

Purpose To control rolling through the spine with your abdominals.

Watchpoints • Keep your eyes focused on your knees so that the head does not touch the mat. • Keep the shoulders sliding down the back. • Keep the heels close to the body. • Sink the navel into the spine to lead with the lower back. • Use the momentum of the exhale to help you come up.

starting position

1. Balance in a C curve, leaning just back of your sitz bones.
2. Relax your hands on your shins, feet close to the buttocks. Shoulders slide down the back; the gaze is toward the knees (fig. 4.18). Try to keep your toes off the floor unless you are doing the modification.

movement 1

1. Inhale to drop the navel into the spine and roll back (fig. 4.19).
2. Exhale to return forward.
3. Repeat six to eight times.

movement 2

1. Inhale to drop the navel into the spine and roll slightly back off your sitz bones (fig. 4.20).
2. Exhale to return, keeping the body in a C curve. If

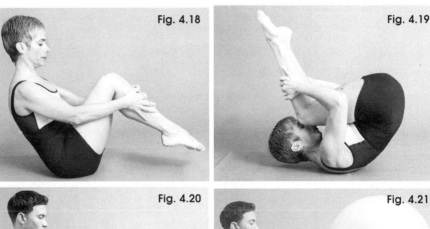

Fig. 4.18

Fig. 4.19

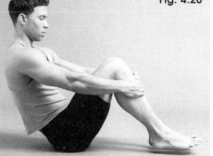

Fig. 4.20

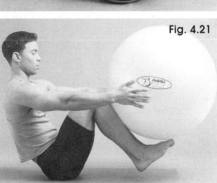

Fig. 4.21

necessary, keep the feet on the floor and work on dropping the navel to scoop the abdominals and feel the C curve.

3. Add the ball when you have mastered the technique and rhythm of rolling back (fig. 4.21).

the rules when legs come up

When the legs are raised up into the air, to protect the lower back we sink it into the mat. Think of sliding the ribs slightly closer to the pelvis rather than forcing the lower back down and causing tension in the spinal muscles.

You can check whether you have done this by being sure that you cannot fit your fingers between the small of your back and the mat. If you lower your legs too close to the mat in exercises such as Single or Double Leg Stretch, your lower back may pop up and arch. This strains the back. The stronger the abdominals become, the lower you can take the legs without lifting the lower back.

Single Leg Stretch

For the following exercises we are taking the legs into the air so the pelvis moves out of neutral and into a position in which the lower back is imprinted or flattened onto the mat. Single Leg Stretch is a great abdominal exercise. If you have neck tension do not use the ball and leave the head on the mat. If you have lower back pain keep the legs higher than a 45-degree angle as you extend them.

Purpose To work on coordination, breathing, and abdominal strength.
Watchpoints • If you have neck tension leave your head down on the mat for the entire exercise and do not use the ball. • Keep ankles, knees, and hips in alignment. • Keep legs fully stretched, toes softly pointed. • The upper torso is stable; shoulder blades slide down the back. • Hollow the abdominals, being sure that the lower back is resting fully on the mat. • Eye gaze is on the thighs, not the ceiling.

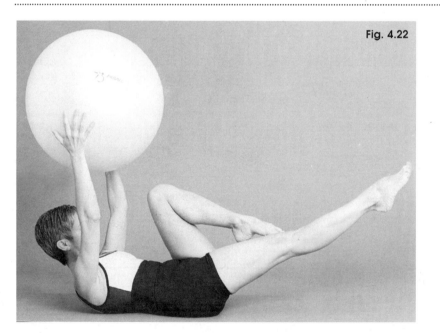

Fig. 4.22

starting position
Lie flat on your back, knees to chest. Hold the ball on your knees.

movement
1. Inhale to prepare, holding the ball in the air above you.
2. Exhale to bring the chin toward your chest as you simultaneously extend one leg 45 degrees from the floor (fig. 4.22).
3. Inhale to switch legs.
4. Exhale to stretch out the other leg 45 degrees from the floor.
5. Inhale to switch, and exhale to extend the leg.
6. Repeat five sets, or ten times with each leg.

Double Leg Stretch

The following is a graceful yet powerful exercise to build the powerhouse. There is a flow and control between the stretching out of the limbs and the tight ball position in between. Don't forget the marriage of breath and movement. The extra weight of the ball makes this a supreme abdominal tightener. Keep your legs high if you have lower back pain.

Purpose To build the abdominals and coordination. To practice linking breath with movement.

Watchpoints • If you have neck tension, keep the head on the mat and do not use the ball. • Keep your navel-to-spine connection to imprint the lower back onto the mat. • Be sure that the arms extend straight alongside and up from the ears. • Legs are parallel and connected; toes are long. • In movement 2, keep the eye gaze on the thighs, not the ceiling. Try not to let the head pull forward. • Do not let your legs drop so low that your lower back arches off the mat. • Do not hunch the shoulders.

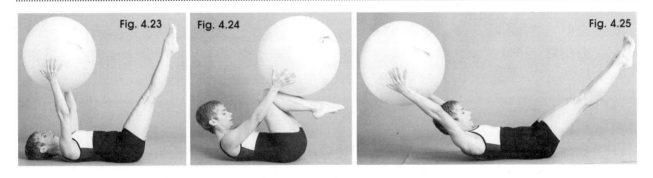

Fig. 4.23   Fig. 4.24   Fig. 4.25

starting position

1. Pull your legs into your chest.
2. Hold the ball on your knees or ankles.
3. Lengthen the back of the neck.

movement 1: leave head on mat

1. Inhale to extend legs and arms, with arms just above the head, legs 45 degrees or higher from the ground (fig. 4.23).
2. Exhale to bring the ball to your ankles.
3. Inhale to stretch legs and arms.
4. Exhale to fold into a ball.
5. Repeat six to eight times.

movement 2: lift head—intermediate

1. Inhale to prepare.
2. Exhale to curl into a ball, chin to chest, hands on the side of the ball (fig. 4.24).
3. Inhale to extend legs and arms, arms just behind the head, legs 45 degrees from the floor (fig. 4.25).
4. Exhale to bring the ball to your ankles.
5. Inhale to stretch legs and arms. Exhale to fold into a ball.
6. Repeat six to eight times.

Obliques

You will really feel this one, as it targets the obliques and we do not use these crisscrossing abdominals as much as the others. Place the ball between your knees, pulling it slightly forward to keep it in place. Squeezing the ball between the legs targets the inner thighs and the muscles deep in the pelvic floor. Try to do this exercise slowly and precisely, keeping the pelvis in neutral. With each exhale think of sliding the rib cage toward the opposite hipbone.

Purpose To target the oblique muscles and the inner thighs.
Watchpoints • Hands are loosely clasped behind the head; elbows are wide.
• Keep the tailbone down on the mat and try not to rock the pelvis. • Keep the abdominals flat and hollowed.

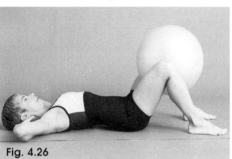

Fig. 4.26

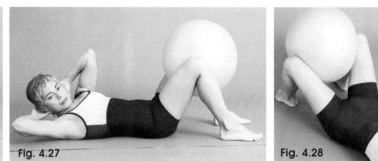

Fig. 4.27

Fig. 4.28

starting position

Lie on your back with the ball positioned between your knees. Feet remain flat on the mat. Hands are behind the head, elbows wide (fig. 4.26).

movement 1: obliques twist

1. Inhale to prepare.
2. Exhale to curl your upper body, chin to chest.
3. Inhale stay. Exhale to bring the left rib cage across the body as you squeeze the ball (fig. 4.27).
4. Inhale to center, chin to chest.
5. Exhale to bring the right rib cage across the body as you squeeze the ball.
6. Repeat eight times on each side.

movement 2: just squeeze

1. Keep your head on the mat. Inhale to slightly release the ball.
2. Exhale to squeeze the ball hard, isolating the inner thighs (fig. 4.28).
3. Repeat six to eight times.

The Rollover

When I first learned this exercise it was positioned near the beginning of the workout, when I did not feel warmed-up enough to do it. It is definitely a challenging exercise, a highly controlled movement, and a wonderful finish to the abdominal series—if you are ready for it. Try it first without the ball and think of peeling away from the mat one vertebra at a time, using the abdominals, not the arms, to lift the legs overhead. Do not take your weight so far back that you are crunching back onto your neck. Keep your head aligned on your spine; if necessary, place a cushion under your hips to aid you.

Purpose To strengthen the abdominals and improve flexibility in the lower back and hamstrings.

Watchpoints • Keep your arms on the floor and avoid using the hands to help you get the legs overhead—use the abdominals. • Keep your navel-to-spine connection. • Keep your head aligned on the spine and do not take your weight too far back onto your neck.

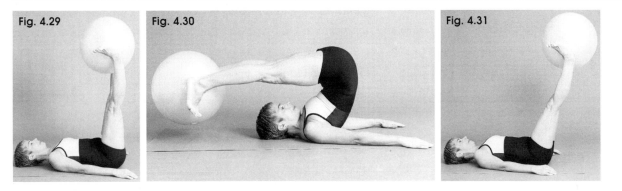

Fig. 4.29   Fig. 4.30   Fig. 4.31

starting position

1. Lie on your back with your arms at your side, palms on the mat.
2. Pick the ball up between your ankles, bend the knees, and extend your legs to the ceiling at a 90-degree angle to the floor (fig. 4.29).

movement

1. Inhale to prepare.
2. Exhale to peel away from the mat while extending the legs overhead.
3. Inhale to touch the ball to floor and then lift so that legs are parallel to the floor (fig. 4.30).

4. Exhale to roll through the spine one vertebra at a time.
5. Lower the ball to an angle at which you are able to keep your lower back on the mat (fig. 4.31).
6. Repeat five times.

If the Pilates on the Ball abdominal exercises are crucial to the health of the back, then so are the extensions. The extension exercises detailed in the next chapter complement the abdominal exercises by opening up the spine and creating space between the vertebrae. Extensions on the ball also challenge the large superficial muscles of the trunk and legs in addition to the small deep muscles close to the spine. Good back fitness does not mean a rigid spine; extensions promote spinal flexibility as well as strength.

5
The Extensions

An Average Sunday: My Story

It is an average Sunday, a day off. I wake early. My eyes jolt open, my mind already jostling with ideas, plans, needs, desires. Relax, I tell myself. It's Sunday. But wild horses cannot keep me still. In fact it is with the manic surge of wild horses that I bound from bed, tug on my clothes, and bang my elbow on the edge of the dresser, barely registering the pain. One thought I have is about the backyard. It is the dead of winter, the ground is frozen under six inches of snow, but I want to be, *have* to be, outside. I pull on my boots, yank on my coat. It is 8 A.M.—my day off—and already I'm in a race against time.

In the backyard I stomp around taking measurements, too swift to be accurate. I come back inside, make coffee, and have a new elated thought. I need a drafting ruler and tear open the junk drawer to look for one. The drawer is a mess. Impulsively I take everything out, determined to set it in order. The hammer and the paint-can opener belong in the basement. As I take them downstairs I remember that the kitchen wall needs painting. Today I could do it—I have the energy to do it. Why not walk to the paint store, stuff the quart can in my knapsack, and return home with the paint on my back?

Meanwhile what did I come downstairs to do? I bound back upstairs thinking, that's it: I want hedges, not fences; and I pull on my boots to go outside to remeasure. Once in the backyard I suddenly remember that I need to put in two more paving stones to complete the path I started last fall. I hurl myself to the shed, half flying: truly, I am barely able to keep my feet on the ground. Flinging open the shed door, I rip out the shovel and stop dead in my tracks. I am furious: the ground is frozen!

Does this manic dance sound like the beginnings of a breakdown? Do I truly believe I can fly? My doctor suggests Ritalin to bring my body and my mind to rest. But I have always refused. As a friend once said to me, why take drugs when you can spin through life six steps ahead of everyone else? Thankfully I have learned to use exercise—and breath—to tranquilize my manic dance.

Be Balanced, Be Sane

Extensions on the ball are about torso strength, balance, and a profound feeling of opening up the body. Balance is what is needed when we get on a stepladder to remove a can of soup from a top shelf or to keep ourselves on kilter after swinging a golf club. Balance is also what is needed to combat the chronic restlessness, impulsiveness, and anxiety that are symptomatic of our time.

Balance in our physical world can also transfer to our emotional and spiritual worlds. This is why the yogis teach balancing postures. Practicing postures that challenge equilibrium reconnects us with our inner peace and strength. Not only do we experience a physical exertion when we attempt to hold the Tree or Warrior posture, but the sense of balance has a profound effect on our well-being. At no time in our histories have we needed this more. As we move into the new millennium there is no sign of things slowing down, of the perpetual motion letting up. We desperately need to make a detour, take a slower path, and restore harmony in our lives, and we know it. Many of us are now convinced that the key to mental and physical health is balance—balance between inner and outer, visible and invisible, doing and not doing.

We also need to find balance between what we can accomplish and what we cannot. Sometimes we do fall. We cannot, no matter what our perfectionist hearts believe, control everything. The unexpected occurs: the surface under a foot, a surface we have stepped on many times before, suddenly gives way. Or we find ourselves in an automobile accident, our legs and arms flying as we lurch inside the stationary structure of the car's steel frame. Thankfully most situations in life where we lose balance are not as traumatic or life threatening. However, they can sting emotionally if we allow the humiliation of falling to affect us.

As we get older we become more and more afraid of falling and usually avoid challenging activities. The more we avoid these activities, the more our balancing skills diminish. Working on a mobile ball raises the stakes of balance in a way that few exercise methods do. In a fifty-minute workout the ball will drift and you may roll off. But is this the end of the world? Remember how as a child you fell often and hardly recalled the physical pain or the humiliation. You are not going to skin your knees or chin doing these ball exercises, but you will improve your coordination and teach yourself to make the split-second adjustments needed to avoid a fall. And if you do tumble, you will practice falling with safety and grace. The ball can be used at any age to safely develop balancing skills.

Extension versus Flexion

Not only are many of us discouraged by failures, exhausted by the chaos of our unbalanced lives, and fearful of falling, but we spend a disproportionate amount of time curling our spines forward. Take a moment to count up the hours per day you spend collapsed in front of a computer or over the steering wheel of your car. Our spines—and our hearts—have forgotten how to do the carefree backbends of a child. We desperately need to balance the flexion of our lives, the closing off of the body, with extension, an opening up of the body.

In the previous chapters we learned how the extensor muscles of the back work alongside the abdominals to create a strong inner core. When the abdominal powerhouse and the postural muscles are well trained the body is ready for safe spinal extensions as well as hefty, outer movements of the legs and the arms. Extensions on the ball strengthen not only the spine but also the back of the legs and the arms too. The goal is to have the abdominal powerhouse perfectly still and contracted while the legs or arms are moving.

After any extension exercise it is crucial to stretch out the spine with flexion—exercises that fold your body forward. If extensions invigorate and empower us with expansion, flexion folds us inward to a place of calm and serenity. Flexion releases the spine, especially the muscles in the lower back, and, in some positions, allows the hamstrings to relax and stretch. Shell on the Ball or Shell on the Mat are luxurious counterposes to extension.

The Extension Exercises

Extensions can aggravate lower back pain if they are not done with attentive care. If you have lower back or sciatic nerve problems or scoliosis be cautious and keep the movement very small.

Let's review the rules when extending the spine.
- Elongate slowly. Do not arch up; at first you may come up only a few inches.
- Remember the navel-to-spine connection and pull the abdominals up into the spine.

- Do not shorten the neck at the top of the movement. Keep the head aligned, eye gaze straight ahead or on the mat, depending on the position of the body.

- Elongate the spine when coming down; do not collapse down.

- Stretch the spine afterward in flexion.

The Swan

The Swan's emphasis is on elongating—not arching—the spine and the ball allows for more range of motion than on the mat. Those with lower back pain must keep this movement very small. Be sure that your abdominals are working to support the lower back. Movement 1 helps you practice lifting the belly button up and into the spine. Notice how on the exhale the abdominal muscles engage naturally.

Purpose To extend the spine. To review the navel-to-spine connection.
Watchpoints • Keep the shoulder blades sliding down. • Keep the back of the neck long. • Keep the elbows close to the body. • The back of the legs should remain straight at all times. • Plant your toes for balance.

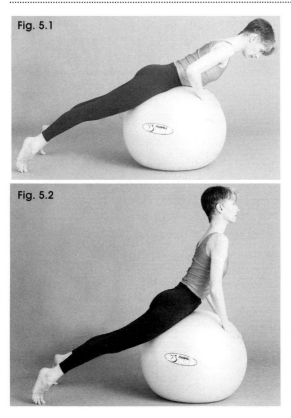

Fig. 5.1

Fig. 5.2

starting position

1. Kneel behind the ball.
2. Climb on the ball and drop your pelvis weight onto the ball.
3. Plant your toes on the floor and be sure that your legs are straight, just wider than shoulder-distance apart.
4. Place your index fingers and thumbs in a diamond shape on the front top of the ball.

movement 1

1. Plant your toes and lift your head just higher than horizontal, so there is a long line from the crown of the head to the toes. Eye gaze is on the floor (fig. 5.1).
2. Inhale to slide your shoulder blades down, keeping your torso parallel to the ground.
3. Exhale to lift the navel up and off the ball.
4. Inhale to drop the navel.
5. Exhale to lift the navel.
6. Repeat five times.

movement 2

1. Start with your head and upper body just higher than horizontal to the ground.
2. Inhale to slide your shoulder blades down. Tighten your abdominal muscles. Eye gaze is on the floor (fig. 5.1).
3. Exhale to slowly lift your upper body, pressing your hips into the ball (fig. 5.2).
4. Inhale at the top of the ball.
5. Exhale to return to starting position.
6. Repeat four to six times.

63

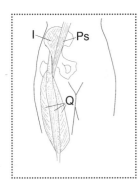

anatomy on the ball: leg muscles

The hip flexors—the psoas and iliacus—are some of the strongest muscles in the body. The long psoas muscle originates on the lower spine and crosses in front of the pelvis to insert on the top of the thighbone. The psoas is the major hip flexor of the body. The iliacus originates on the rim of the pelvis; it is an important deep muscle that helps support and stabilize the pelvis.

The quadriceps are massive muscles on the front of the legs. Known informally as the quads, they consist of four separate muscles that straighten the leg and stabilize the knee. The quads are the strongest muscles in the body.

Swan Dive

The following extension is more advanced than the ordinary Swan but will benefit your entire body if you are ready for it. Avoid movement 2 if you have lower back pain; instead keep the hands on the ball (movement 1) and keep the knees bent the entire time to take the pressure off the lower back. Remember to work at your own pace; you do not have to look like the photographs here. Pull up your abdominals, breathe deeply, and let your energy soar.

Purpose To strengthen the back muscles and the backs of the legs.

Watchpoints • If you have lower back pain keep the knees bent the entire time and stick with movement 1. • Do not overarch the neck. Keep the back of the neck long and open. • Keep the abdominals connected, shoulder blades sliding down throughout the move.

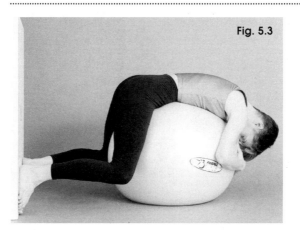

Fig. 5.3

starting position

Relax the body over the front of the ball. Legs are bent and turned out. Balls of the feet are against a wall in the frog position, heels facing each other, toes apart (fig. 5.3). Heels can be apart but take care to keep the toes aligned with the knees.

movement 1: preparation for swan dive

1. Inhale to lengthen out from the crown of the head, hands resting on the ball (fig. 5.4). This is the dive position. The back of the legs should now be very straight.

2. Exhale to bend your knees and lift your chest toward the ceiling, hands on the ball (fig. 5.5). Your pelvis will push into the ball and your body weight will stop the ball from rolling out from under you.

3. Inhale to lengthen the spine in the dive position, straightening the legs, hands on the ball (fig. 5.4).

4. Exhale to bend the knees and lift the chest toward the ceiling (fig. 5.5).

5. Inhale to lengthen the spine in the dive position, straightening the legs (fig. 5.4).

6. Exhale to bend the knees and relax the body over the ball to the starting position (fig. 5.3).

7. Repeat this sequence two or three times.

movement 2: *full swan dive—intermediate*

1. Avoid this movement if you have lower back pain. Inhale to lengthen the spine as you reach the arms out long overhead, shoulder-distance apart, palms down (fig. 5.6). This is the dive position. The backs of the legs should now be very straight.
2. Exhale to bend the knees and lift the chest toward the ceiling, opening the arms (fig. 5.7).

3. Inhale to lengthen the spine in the dive position, straightening the legs (fig. 5.6).
4. Exhale to bend the knees and lift the chest toward the ceiling, opening the arms (fig. 5.7).
5. Inhale to lengthen the spine in the dive position, straightening the legs (fig. 5.6).
6. Exhale to bend the knees and relax the body over the ball to the starting position (fig. 5.3).
7. Repeat this sequence twice.

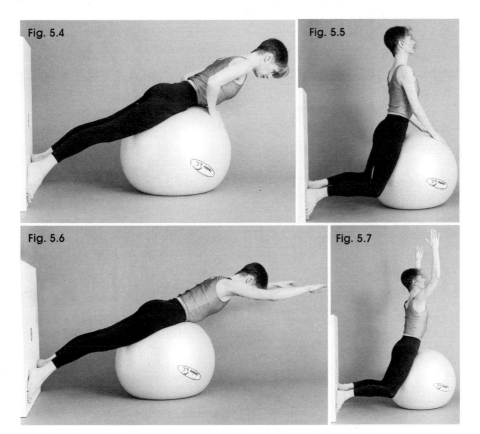

Fig. 5.4

Fig. 5.5

Fig. 5.6

Fig. 5.7

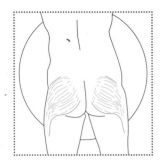

anatomy on the ball: more leg muscles

Muscles of the posterior hip are the gluteals, or glutes. These are the buttock muscles that work with the external hip rotators to create motion at the hip joint and stabilize the pelvis while walking or moving the legs.

Gluteus maximus, pictured above, is the big meaty muscle of the buttock. It is a major hip extensor and it rotates the leg outward. The gluteus medius originates from the top side rim of the pelvis and runs down to the top side of the thighbone. It abducts the hip (moves the hip away from the body in the frontal plane). The gluteus minimus is a small muscle just in front of the medius. It abducts the thigh and rotates the leg inward.

Shell on the Ball

After the Swans you need to ease out the lower back. Remember to initiate the movement with the abdominals. If rolling up on the ball feels too scary at first, do the Shell on the Mat (see chapter 8). If you are comfortable doing Shell on the Ball, you can make the exercise more challenging by introducing the element of speed. With quick, concise movements exhale up into the Shell and inhale down into the plank.

Purpose To stretch out the spine after extension. To practice balance and coordination.

Watchpoints • Avoid the Shell on the Ball if you have knee injuries.
• Make sure the ball is directly in front of the knees each time (plank position) or you will not be in the right position when you roll into the Shell.

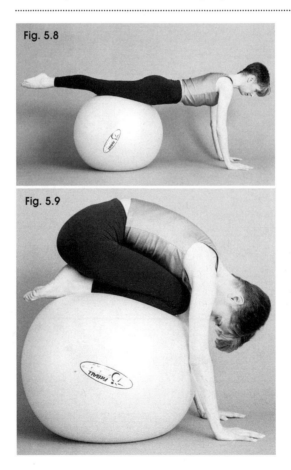

Fig. 5.8

Fig. 5.9

starting position

1. Kneel in front of your ball.
2. Crawl over the ball and walk out so that the hands are directly below the shoulders and the ball is directly in front of the knees (plank position) (fig. 5.8).
3. Squeeze the thighs together and keep the sides of the knees touching each other.

movement

1. Inhale to lengthen through the spine.
2. Exhale to bend the knees and hips and let the ball roll under you, leaving the hands firmly planted where they are on the mat (fig. 5.9).
3. Inhale as you stay in the Shell.
4. Exhale to roll down into the plank position, making sure the ball is just in front of your knees.
5. Repeat three or four times. During the last repetition remain in the Shell for a few breaths.

More Extensions

These are challenging torso exercises that strengthen the glutes and hamstrings, shape your legs, tone your abdominals, and strengthen your arms and wrists. You work the entire torso as the center of gravity continuously changes.

Purpose To strengthen the glutes, hamstrings, abdominals, and back extensor muscles.

Watchpoints • Do not overarch the lower back. • Be sure that the body is rocked forward and stays in the long bow shape. • Distribute weight evenly between both hands. • Do not allow the abdominals to drop or the hips to droop. • Lower the head between your arms but keep the head aligned on the spine, the back of the neck long.

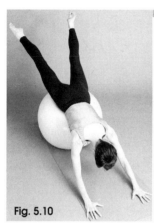 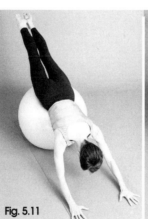 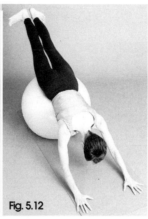

Fig. 5.10   Fig. 5.11   Fig. 5.12

starting position

1. Kneel in front of the ball.
2. Crawl over the ball and walk out so that the hands are directly below the shoulders and the ball rolls down the body onto the thighs (see fig. 5.8).
3. Without moving the hands, pitch the body forward, bending the elbows slightly and lifting the feet. The ball will roll under the pelvis to support the body (see "Grasshopper" on next page, fig. 5.14).

movement 1: open and close legs

1. Inhale to open the legs shoulder-distance apart (fig. 5.10).
2. Exhale to squeeze legs together, keeping the body in a long bow shape (fig. 5.11).
3. Inhale to open the legs. Exhale to squeeze the legs together.
4. Repeat eight times, keeping the legs very straight.

movement 2: beats

1. Inhale to beat the toes together three times, keeping the toes long and legs straight (fig. 5.11).
2. Exhale to beat the heels together three times, keeping the feet flexed and legs straight (fig. 5.12).
3. Inhale. Inhale. Inhale. (Toe. Toe. Toe.)
4. Exhale. Exhale. Exhale. (Heel. Heel. Heel.)
5. Repeat six times.

Grasshopper

Like many of the extension exercises, the Grasshopper is also adapted from the Pilates Ladder Barrel—a tall barrel used in a Pilates studio to strengthen and stretch the spine and develop the arms and legs. The Grasshopper is a challenging exercise that utilizes body strength, balance, and coordination. Remember: the goal of all these extensions is to stabilize the body at its core while moving the outer limbs. Afterward, remember to stretch out the spine.

Purpose To coordinate breath and movement. To strengthen the glutes, hamstrings, abdominals, and back extensor muscles.

Watchpoints • Try to not let the tops of the legs drop as the ankles cross. • Lift the navel up into the spine to protect the lower back. • Keep shoulder blades sliding down. • Don't let the legs extend wider than shoulder-distance apart.

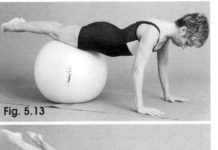

Fig. 5.13

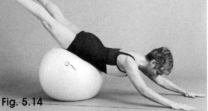

Fig. 5.14

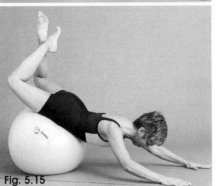

Fig. 5.15

starting position

Crawl over the ball and walk out so that the hands are directly below the shoulders and the thighs rest on the ball (plank position) (fig. 5.13).

movement—intermediate

1. Inhale to slide the shoulder blades down, remaining in the plank position.
2. On the exhale, without moving the hands, pitch the body forward in a long bow shape, bending the elbows slightly and lifting and opening the legs shoulder-distance apart (fig. 5.14). The ball will roll under the pelvis to support the body.
3. Inhale to cross or beat one foot on top of the other three times, keeping the knees as high as you can. Inhale beat, inhale beat, inhale beat (fig. 5.15).
4. Exhale, still pitched forward in the long bow position, to extend your legs up and behind, shoulder-distance apart (fig. 5.14).
5. Inhale to return to starting position (plank position).
6. Repeat three times.
7. To finish, walk your hands back toward the ball and relax over it.

Extensions are designed to expand the body, stretch and align the spine, and make it easier to breathe. Extensions on the ball have the added advantage of toning and strengthening the legs and buttocks while they build core strength and stabilization from the inside out.

In the next chapter you will isolate muscles of the arms, shoulders, feet, calves, and legs and work the outer extremities. Control of the outer, superficial muscles can only occur effectively when the inner muscles are well trained. Now you can test the principle of training from the inside out as you transfer movement and power to the outer muscles of the arms and legs.

6

Pilates on the Ball
Arm- and Footwork

A few well-designed movements, properly performed in a balanced sequence, are worth hours of doing sloppy calisthenics.
—Philip Friedman and Gail Eisen, *The Pilates Method of Physical and Mental Conditioning*

Jenny's Story

Jenny leans deeper over her steering wheel. *Quick, quicker, quickest* purr her windshield wipers as she races into the gym's parking lot. Why is she rushing? She hates the gym—or rather, she tells me, she is unconvinced that the exercises she does there really help her.

When Jenny first telephoned me I asked her to describe her typical workout. She flops on a mat, does twenty to twenty-five obligatory crunches and a few stretches. In her peripheral vision she sees the weight section in the corner of the room and feels guilty because her doctor prescribed weight-bearing exercises to counter the osteoporosis that runs in her family, yet she has never set foot in that part of the gym. She has an image of herself as slim, neat, and feminine, and placing one of those steel and no doubt grimy barbells in her manicured hands goes against every image that she has of herself. A friend encouraged her to try the weight machines instead. "I found the machines cold and impersonal," she told me. "And my chest and arm muscles hurt so much the next day I could hardly steer my car." She didn't want to be in pain, and she didn't want bulky muscles. Worse still, she read somewhere that muscle turns into ugly fat the moment you stop weight training.

I reassured Jenny that she would not bulk up and that muscle did not turn to fat in the way she imagined. Pilates armwork is unique and wonderful, I enthused. It builds long, lean muscles without strain or sweat. She met my eagerness with skepticism, and I did not hear from her for months.

When Jenny finally joined a class it was the result of a difficult business trip. First, in the check-in line she struggled with her carry-on, stuffed to capacity with samples and press kits. Until she could locate a cart she had to kick the bag along with herculean leg kicks, because she could barely pick it up. When she got inside the plane, she looked frantically for a man to help her get the carry-on into the overhead bin. No one helped her; she spent the entire flight with the unwieldy bag stuffed under the seat in front of her. Here she was, forty-five-years old and feeling like an invalid. "That was it," she told me. "If it's not too late to change myself into something stronger, what am I waiting for?"

Physical Fragility Is a Liability

In today's world of slipped disks and computer- and work-related injuries, it is unfair (and unrealistic) for any woman to expect a man or anyone else to carry her load around. Physical fragility is a liability at any age. If we are strong we can do myriad things better. Strength equals independence for senior women. Chores become more manageable; we can get in and out of cars, lift groceries overhead, and pick up grandbabies. For young and middle-aged women, pulling your own weight helps protect against work-related strains. It builds confidence, too.

There are often psychological obstacles that keep women from strength training, though these barriers are breaking down in recent years. When I work with a student such as Jenny who is very reluctant to try weight train-ing, I find it essential to address her opposition and concerns before commit-ting to using weights, even small weights. For some women it is a question of aesthetics—do they want a muscular arm or not? Other women need to work through the emotional baggage of growing up as a member of the "weaker sex," and this takes time. Jan Todd describes how physical fragility can lead to a lack of confidence in other parts of one's life. "I see friends in their forties pushing away from life, not trying things," says Todd, an historian and strong-woman, to *Health* interviewer Ann Japenga in the November/December 1999 issue, adding: "The physicality of my life taught me not to be afraid."

Even though she may not, like Todd, end up in the Guinness Book of World Records as the world's strongest woman, a female trainer's own attitude and enthusiasm for weights can be contagious and can greatly influence her students. Pilates on the Ball armwork is a wonderful way for women to be introduced to weights as well as helping those who are already using weights add variety and *meaning* to their workout. *Meaning* is also why this unusual armwork is beneficial for men.

71

Inside Out: Benefits for Men and Women

Traditional weight training usually works from the outside in, isolating and developing the large superficial peripheral muscles of the arms and legs, often to the detriment of shoulder, upper body, hip, and leg flexibility. Yet working from the inside out is a safer way to keep the muscles balanced. The small, deep postural muscles and the musculature of the powerhouse build a strong core to support the outer muscles effectively. The theory of inside out teaches men and women how to utilize their entire bodies and connect with their core to help prevent lower back pain and potential injuries.

Pilates on the Ball arm- and footwork is functional training, not simply weight lifting. Functional training means that the exercises relate directly to the activities you perform in your daily life, such as going up and down stairs, lifting a soup can from a shelf, or getting in and out of chairs. Even though we seem to be isolating muscles as in a traditional weight program, this arm- and footwork helps you to focus on the movements as a whole. Sitting tall on the ball, standing on the feet, pressing the ball against the wall, or using the ball as a weight bench are comfortable, efficient ways to train the body as a unit, not simply isolate, overuse, or bulk up muscles.

Resistance = Bone Workout

When it comes to your bone and muscle health there is bad news and good news. Unfortunately, unless the muscles are challenged the body will break down muscle tissue and lose strength and bone density as you age. This process can begin as early as age twenty-one! The good news is that it is never too late to begin to strengthen and tone muscles. The most effective way to do so is by adding resistance. Adding resistance to your workout not only improves muscular strength and endurance but also helps to stabilize the muscles in their joints.

Working out with a few light weights two or three times a week builds strong bones and can help you lose weight. Adding resistance raises your metabolic rate so that long after you have left your ball or set down your weights you continue to burn calories. Resistance training also helps to combat osteoporosis, the silent bone-stealing disease that mainly affects women. Recent research argues that resistance training can begin at any age, even eighty and up, and be highly effective.

Another incentive for performing weight work is muscle definition. Unless women and men take up weights, as they age they lose muscle tone fast. The wonderful thing about Pilates armwork is that no matter how out of shape you are, you will see results fast. Here we use only one- or two-pound weights.

Small weights are easier to control, and they build the long, lean muscles for which Pilates-obsessed dancers and movie stars are famous.

Recent studies also document the benefits of resistance training in individuals with heart and other health problems. One study found that unfit women who began weight training three times a week decreased blood cholesterol levels by almost 10 percent. A recent American Heart Association survey, published in the journal *Circulation*, found that lifting weights is highly beneficial for reducing blood pressure and body fat and improving glucose metabolism and cardiovascular function. "Resistance training offers significant benefits to health and fitness beyond the cutting and shaping of muscles," said Dr. Barry A. Franklin, an author of the study. Weight lifting, he said, could benefit some patients who had heart attacks because "if muscles are stronger a person's heart rate and blood pressure response will be lower, creating less demand on the heart when something is lifted."

Joseph Pilates himself designed specific pieces of equipment, machines with pulleys and springs, to add resistance to his matwork. Most of the arm- and footwork exercises I've selected for this chapter are adapted from pieces of equipment found in most Pilates studios. Weights and your ball are two practical, comfortable ways to add resistance.

Precision and Pace

In Pilates on the Ball we are training the muscles to move the limbs through space with precision and economy. We are striving for accuracy of movement, which equals economy of movement. We desire no extra movement than is necessary and no unwanted strain.

Since a lot can go wrong when you stand upon your feet and bear weight, you may want to check yourself in a mirror as you approach the footwork. Keep an even pace as you go through the various foot positions; the aim is to build stamina without overdeveloping one area. Exaggerated knee bends or deep squats will stress joints and aggravate misalignment of feet, ankles, and knees. Instead try for smaller, controlled movements where your object is to work the small muscles around the knee as well as strengthen the large quad muscles and inner and outer thighs. We are striving for half a dozen precise movements rather than two dozen sloppy or jerky ones.

Even though there are rest periods or breathers placed throughout other parts of the workout, with this arm- and footwork, unlike traditional weight work, we do not need to rest between sets. A continuous pace, supported by good technique, fatigues and tones muscles and builds endurance without strain.

why don't I feel sore after Pilates armwork?

The principle of traditional weight training is to use heavy weights to overload muscles by working them to fatigue. Afterward soreness can be felt in the large muscles as they recover.

In Pilates armwork the aim is not to isolate a muscle into exhaustion. Remember: we use only one- or two-pound weights. Small weights do not break down muscle tissue or stress joints. The position that the arm is in when you lift the small weights, and the fact that you are moving the arms through different planes, contributes to the effectiveness of the movement.

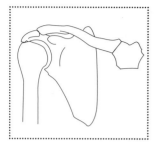

anatomy on the ball: the shoulder

The shoulder girdle is a complex, highly mobile structure, with the shoulder blades in back and collarbone in front. Notice that the shoulder blades are attached to the trunk only in one place: where the collarbone meets with the sternum. This is why there is so much movement in the shoulder joint and why isolated arm movements are possible.

The shoulder joint is much more exposed than the hip joint; thus, shoulder dislocations are common. This joint moves as a ball and socket as well as a hinge. Notice too that the upper arm (humerus) and forearm (radius and ulna) move freely, as do the hands and fingers.

The Armwork

Sitting on the ball while you perform the armwork is especially helpful for those with tightness in the hips and lower back. The ball will allow you to sit tall and operate the body efficiently. Try not to let the ribs protrude or "pop out"; soften the ribs by thinking of their connection to the abdominals and by filling the back rib cage with air.

As you perform the exercises make sure that the lower back is in neutral pelvis, neither totally flattened nor in an exaggerated curve. A mirror may help you resolve this. Sometimes the simple act of pulling the navel to the spine will place the pelvis in neutral.

Try the arm exercises first to make sure you have good alignment and technique before adding weights. Are your shoulders rolling forward? Is your collarbone elevated on one side? Is the head straight? Remember that the head is heavy and must be structurally supported. Don't forget about the abdominal connection each and every time you move. Remember this connection when you are not with your ball and weights, for a strong powerhouse will save your back when lifting heavy objects.

Start with one-pound weights and build to two when you can master good alignment and technique with the smaller weights. Heavy weights create strong, well-developed arms but not light, flexible ones. Small weights help you focus on technique, posture, and breathing without straining the body.

Try to keep your shoulder blades, or scapulas, sliding down the back during the armwork. This downward motion should happen without forcing the shoulder blades down or squeezing them together. If the scapulas are not stabilized the small muscles of the rotator cuff are strained.

Do not merely float the arms through space. Try and add resistance to the small weights. Imagine that you are moving thirty pounds of weight through space instead of merely one pound. Mari Winsor refers to this in *The Pilates Powerhouse* as moving the body through wet cement: "The cement prevents you from moving quickly. Because you can't throw your limbs, you have to really concentrate on how the body gets from point A to point B." Adding a certain tension within the muscles as you move the limbs (with or without weights) is a very effective and safe way to build strength without putting stress on tendons and joints.

Using light weights also gives you the time and opportunity to fully expand the muscles as well as fully contract them. You are working the muscles concentrically, contracting or shortening them, as well as eccentrically, extending or expanding them, and both sides of the movement require equal attention.

Work slowly and smoothly through the full range of movement. Focus on the muscle you are attempting to work. Work in healthy alignment. Don't forget to breathe.

Hug a Tree

If you have round shoulders skip Hug a Tree. Forward shoulders indicate that the top of the arm bone rolls inward and that the chest muscles, or pectorals, are short and tight. The next exercise, Open Shoulders, will stretch the pectorals. Another very effective way to stretch the pectorals is to lie back on your ball in the Tabletop with your arms open in a T shape (see chapter 8). Let your small weights gently open the body. With rounded shoulders it is beneficial to strengthen the midback and lower trapezius muscles of the back. Most of the following arm exercises do that.

Purpose To strengthen pectoral muscles. To tone arm muscles.
Watchpoints • Keep tall through the spine with the eyes gazing straight ahead, not on the floor. • Keep shoulder blades sliding down the back. • Don't let the arms open too wide to the side and don't allow the rib cage to pop open. • Make sure the elbows stay lifted. • Keep the abdominal connection.

rib cage placement

Rib cage placement is a crucial part of correct alignment. It is easy for the rib cage to expand or "pop out" when lifting the arms and performing armwork. Try not to allow the rib cage to lift upward or collapse downward. Instead, let the ribs soften into the abdominals while remaining very tall through the spine.

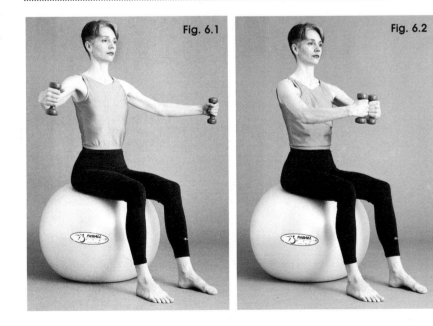

Fig. 6.1   Fig. 6.2

starting position
1. Sit on the center of your ball, knees over ankles, legs just wider than hip-distance apart, feet parallel.
2. Pull navel up and into the back of the spine.

movement
1. Inhale to open arms to the side, keeping the hands in your peripheral vision (fig. 6.1).
2. Exhale to circle the arms together as if around a thick tree. Try to keep the shoulders back and not let them round forward (fig. 6.2).
3. Inhale to open the arms to the side.
4. Exhale to circle the arms together at heart level.
5. Repeat six to eight times.

75

Open Shoulders and Biceps Curls

Small weights will make you strong but will not stress the joints. Remember: navel-to-spine. Try to keep the body steady and perform the moves without moving the head.

Purpose Movement 1 stretches and strengthens the pectorals. Movement 2 strengthens the biceps.

Watchpoints • In biceps curls keep the elbows stiff and in the Tabletop.
• Shoulders blades are sliding down the back at all times.

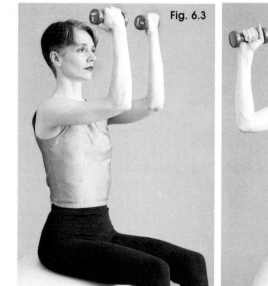
Fig. 6.3

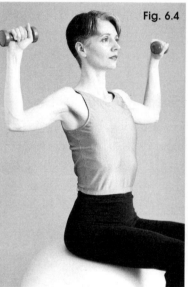
Fig. 6.4

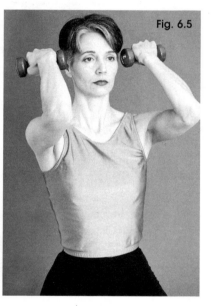
Fig. 6.5

starting position

Sit on the center of your ball, knees over ankles, legs just wider than hip-distance apart, feet parallel.

movement 1: open shoulders

1. Arms are bent and in front of your shoulders, shoulder blades are sliding down the back (fig. 6.3).
2. Inhale to open the arms to the sides (fig. 6.4).
3. Exhale to return.
4. Repeat six to eight times.

movement 2: biceps curls

1. Place elbows high as if on a tabletop, shoulders down.
2. Inhale to open the arms to the front.
3. Exhale to pull weights in by your ears (fig. 6.5).
4. Repeat six to eight times.

Salute

With this exercise you are trying to isolate the triceps, which are at the back of your upper arms. Shoulder blades should remain down as the arms extend upward.

Purpose To strengthen triceps and shoulder stabilizers.

Watchpoints • Keep elbows in a fixed position as you extend your arms; they should point outward slightly. • Avoid hyperextending or locking arms at the top. • Check to be sure that the neck is long and the shoulders are sliding down the back.

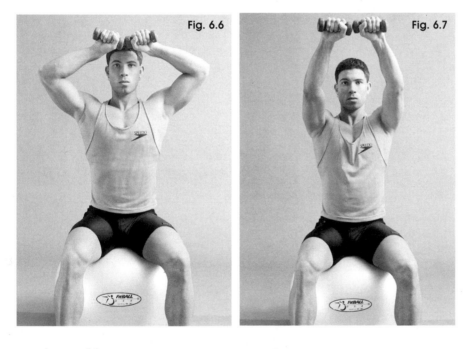

Fig. 6.6   Fig. 6.7

starting position

1. Sit on the center of your ball, knees over ankles, legs just wider than hip-distance apart, feet parallel.
2. Lift arms up to the forehead (fig. 6.6) or, if you are able to keep the shoulder blades in place, to the back of the head.

movement

1. Inhale to prepare.
2. Exhale to extend the arms straight up, keeping the weights close together at the top (fig. 6.7).
3. Inhale to bring the weights to the forehead. Exhale to extend the arms.
4. Repeat six to eight times.

Rowing

This exercise creates full mobility in the ball and socket as well as strengthens deltoids, pectorals, and the latissimus dorsi. It is important to be very aware of the shoulder blades in all arm exercises; this one teaches you to keep the motion small to maintain stabilization of the shoulders.

Purpose To strengthen deltoids and create mobility in the ball and socket.

Watchpoint • Keep hands in your peripheral vision rather than taking the weights behind your shoulders.

anatomy on the ball: arm muscles

The deltoid is a bulky muscle on top of the shoulder that raises the upper arm. *Latissimus dorsi,* or lats, means "widest back muscle." This muscle spans a large portion of the back, attaching eventually on the upper arm. The pectorals are the major muscles of the chest.

The two-headed biceps are in the front of the upper arm. When this muscle works the elbow bends and the forearm and hand move toward the shoulder. The triceps are in the back of the upper arm and work to straighten the elbow.

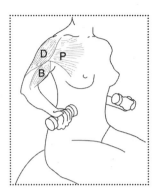

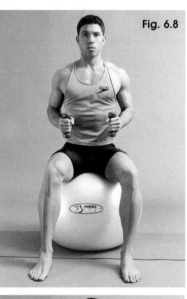

Fig. 6.8

starting position

Sit on the center of your ball, knees over ankles, legs just wider than hip-distance apart, feet parallel. Arms are bent and at the side at waist level (fig. 6.8).

movement

1. Inhale to extend arms forward (fig. 6.9).
2. Exhale to press hands down to the side of the knees (fig. 6.10).
3. Inhale to lift arms as high as possible, keeping the shoulders down (fig. 6.11).

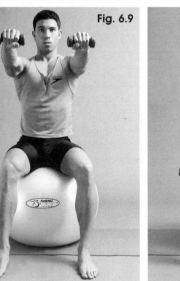

Fig. 6.9

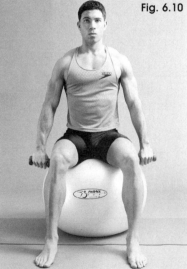

Fig. 6.10

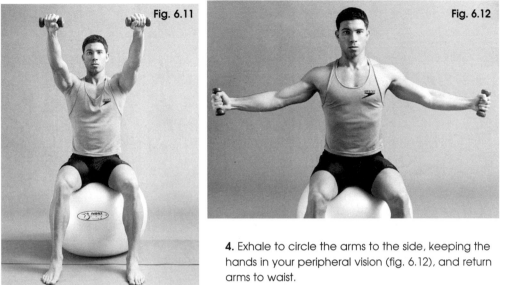

Fig. 6.11

Fig. 6.12

4. Exhale to circle the arms to the side, keeping the hands in your peripheral vision (fig. 6.12), and return arms to waist.
5. Repeat six to eight times.

Flies and More Armwork

If there were ever a sensation of doing exercises on a waterbed this is it. Lying back on your ball you will get a full range of movement, more than on a mat and more comfortable than on a bench press. The ball massages your back as you lift, but the whole body has to work to remain balanced against gravity. Keep the abdominals connected to protect the lower back. Train the shoulder blades to drop down and away from your ears and to remain still during the lifts. Unlike with a stationary weight-training bench, no part of the body can relax on the ball. With this exercise you can use slightly heavier weights (three to five pounds) if desired, because the position of the body, and the arms, can support this.

Purpose Scapula Isolation will warm up the shoulder blades and make you aware of their correct position. Chest Press works the pectorals. Flies work the deltoids and pectorals.

Watchpoints • Make sure your head and neck are totally supported by the ball and not hanging backward. • Keep your weights at heart level and don't let them drift up to head level. • Don't let your buttocks or abdominals sag. • Keep the shoulder blades in place.

79

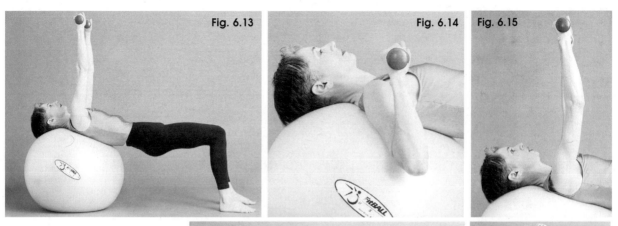

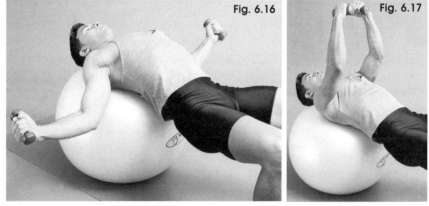

starting position

Sit on your ball. Walk your feet out and carefully let the ball roll under you until your head and neck are totally supported by the ball. Hips are up, abdominals tight.

movement 1: scapula isolation

1. Raise both arms to the ceiling directly above your shoulders.
2. Inhale to lift the arms, raising the tips of the shoulder blades off the ball (fig. 6.13).
3. Exhale to drop the shoulder blades on the ball, keeping arms straight.
4. Repeat five times.

movement 2: chest press

1. Start with weights just above your shoulders (fig. 6.14).
2. Inhale to prepare.
3. Exhale to raise arms, keeping the shoulder blades on the ball (fig. 6.15).
4. Repeat six to eight times.

movement 3: flies

1. Inhale to open your arms to the sides, keeping elbows slightly bent. Hug the ball with the back of your arms (fig. 6.16).
2. Exhale to squeeze your arms together as if around a thick tree, keeping them slightly bent (fig. 6.17).
3. Repeat six to eight times.

The Footwork

Get on your feet now so you can work the buttocks, leg muscles, feet, and ankles. We get a lot of sensory feedback through our feet. The foot contains 26 bones (7 anklebones, 5 instep bones, and 14 toe bones), 31 joints, and 20 muscles. Working in bare feet is the ideal. Often people are locked in the feet. Here is an exercise to help you. Roll a small hard ball under one of your feet. Notice how tension in the foot releases. Roll the ball from the heel of the foot right up to the head of each toe. Don't forget about the three arches—two running lengthwise from heel to ball and one running across the instep. Use a small hard ball to massage your feet whenever they ache.

As mentioned before, a lot can go wrong when you are up on your feet and bearing weight. Make sure you place your feet far enough away from the wall so that when you bend the knees they are positioned directly over the toes without jutting out over the toes. Check yourself against the "knees too far forward" diagram (see sidebar).

As you prepare for the movements, be careful that the tailbone does not roll around the ball. If the tailbone curls around the ball you have lost neutral pelvis. Try to focus on keeping the tailbone heavy and dropped throughout the footwork.

Relax your shoulders as you work. Keep the chin horizontal and the eye gaze straight ahead. The rib cage should be full but not hyperextended. Try the breathing as suggested below; remember you can reverse it if necessary.

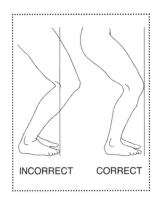

INCORRECT   CORRECT

knees too far forward

Be sure that your feet are far enough away from the wall so that when you bend the knees the lower leg remains vertical and is not too far forward over the toes.

The Footwork Exercises

The distinct positions of the following movements work the feet, ankles, and leg muscles differently. Keep weight equally distributed on both legs and be sure that the knees are in line with the feet. Take care that the feet are not rolling in or out. You are trying to extend the leg muscles fully while being sure that the quadriceps are working to align the kneecap and thighbone. Avoid hyperextending or locking the knees. Remember that the breath can be reversed for all the footwork; you may prefer to inhale to prepare and exhale to bend, rather than the pattern given here.

Purpose To strengthen legs, buttocks, and ankles.

Watchpoints • Don't bend the knees too much. You should be able to see the tips of your toes. • Avoid rolling the ankles in or out and keep the knees aligned over the feet. • In movements 2 and 6 be sure that you are turning out from the hip socket and not the feet. • In the Lower and Lift exercise be sure that the upper body does not move as you are lowering and lifting the heels.

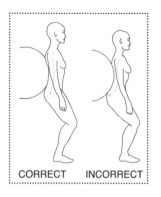

CORRECT   INCORRECT

where is my tailbone?

Be careful that your tailbone does not wrap around the ball. If it does you have lost neutral pelvis. In this footwork you may not go as deeply into the squat as you are used to. Only go as far as you can while still maintaining neutral pelvis.

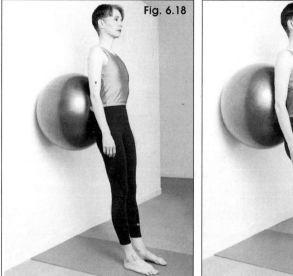

Fig. 6.18

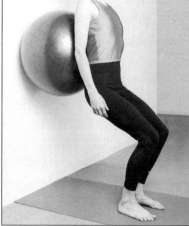

Fig. 6.19

starting position

1. Place the ball against the wall. Stand with heels approximately 20 to 28 inches from the wall, depending on the size of ball.
2. Place the ball at the small curve in the back and press your weight back into the ball. Hands are relaxed at your side; knees are aligned over the feet (fig. 6.18).

movement 1: parallel feet

1. Feet are sitz-bone distance apart and parallel.
2. Inhale to bend the knees, keeping the heels down (fig. 6.19). Make sure that the knees are not too far forward.
3. Exhale to straighten the legs.
4. Repeat six to eight times.

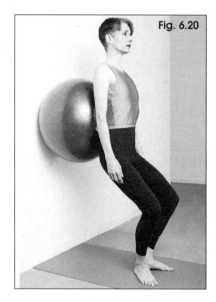

Fig. 6.20

movement 2: small turnout

1. Stand with the toes apart and the heels together in small turnout position.
2. Inhale to bend the knees, keeping the heels down (fig. 6.20).
3. Exhale to straighten the legs.
4. Repeat six to eight times.

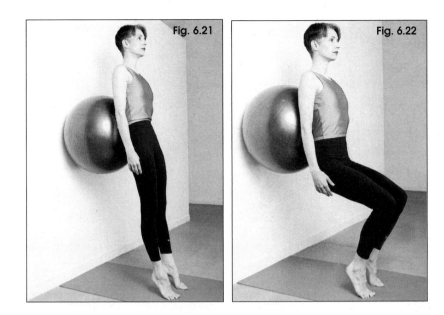

Fig. 6.21
Fig. 6.22

movement 3: high half toe

1. Feet are sitz-bone distance apart and parallel.
2. Lift the heels up high, as if you were wearing high-heeled shoes, and keep them in that position (fig. 6.21).
3. Inhale to bend knees, keeping the heels as high as possible without straining the ankles (fig. 6.22).
4. Exhale to straighten the legs, keeping the heels up.
5. Repeat six to eight times, keeping the heels up.

BodySpheres—Leap Frog

*t*his is a typical BodySpheres move—playful and challenging. You will be springing off the wall onto your arms. Be careful not to jar your shoulders and wrists. Keep your legs and feet aligned as you push off the wall.

With your back to the wall press the front of your pelvis onto the ball. Your knees are bent and your toes are tucked against the bottom edge of the wall. Your arms are pressed against the ball in front of you (fig. 6.23). Inhale to bend the knees deeper. Exhale to push your toes into the wall, then spring forward onto your arms (fig. 6.24). Return to the starting position. Repeat four to six times.

Mari Naumovski notes: This exercise utilizes the push factor in your lower body to propel your upper body through space. Notice the animal quality as you spring from feet to arms in a face-down position.

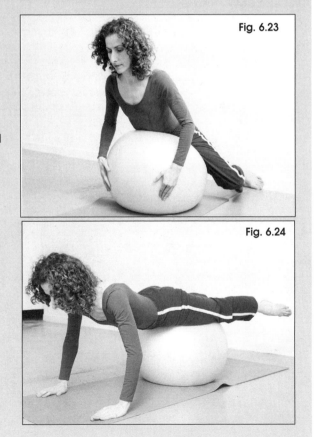

Fig. 6.23
Fig. 6.24

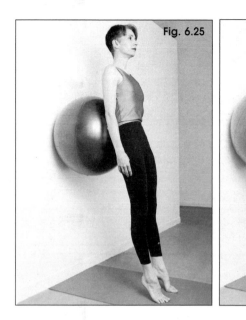

Fig. 6.25

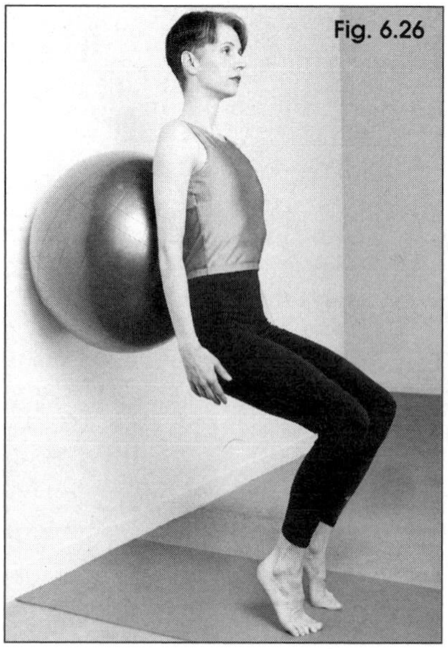

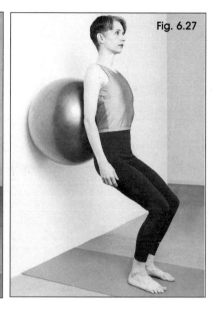

Fig. 6.26

Fig. 6.27

movement 4: lower and lift

1. Feet are sitz-bone distance apart and parallel. Lift the heels up high, as if you were wearing high-heeled shoes (fig. 6.25).
2. Inhale to lower, keeping the heels up (fig. 6.26).
3. Exhale to push the heels down, keeping the knees bent (fig. 6.27).

4. Inhale to lift the heels, keeping the knees bent.
5. Exhale to straighten the legs, keeping the heels up.
6. Inhale to bend the knees, keeping the heels up.
7. Exhale to push the heels down once, keeping the knees bent.
8. Inhale to lift the heels, keeping

the body in the same plane and knees bent.
9. Exhale to lower the heels twice, keeping the knees bent.
10. Inhale to lift the heels, keeping the knees bent.
11. Exhale to straighten the legs.
12. Repeat, building up to five repetitions of this movement sequence.

movement 5: wide squat

1. Begin with feet wider than shoulder-distance apart and slightly turned out (fig. 6.28).
2. Inhale to bend the knees, keeping the heels down. The knees should be aligned over the toes (fig. 6.29).
3. Exhale to stretch the legs.
4. Repeat six to eight times.

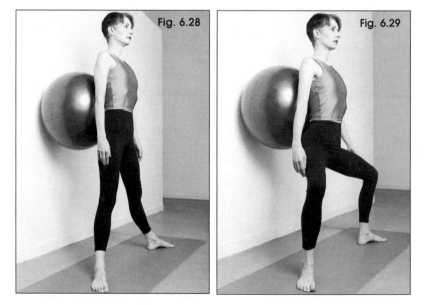

Fig. 6.28

Fig. 6.29

Pilates on the Ball arm- and footwork teaches you to work the upper and lower body efficiently without strain. Yet sometimes no matter how much care you take, how precisely you move your body through space, your body lets you down. Even the healthiest person can have recurring aches and pains. In the next chapter you will work toward rebuilding and restoring the body by using therapeutic and strengthening exercises on the ball. Whether your problems are from a physical weakness, an imbalance, or a trauma, Pilates on the Ball can heal and prevent injuries as well as condition the body while you are recovering from an injury.

7
Restoration and Rebuilding

Susan's Story

When I first met sixty-seven-year-old Susan she had such pain she could barely get out of bed. She had lost almost two inches of height to disintegrating vertebrae and had constant pain from degenerative disk disease. Her rheumatologist told her she was in such bad shape that she wasn't even ready for physiotherapy.

Susan had recently retired from a career as a bookmaker and, in addition to her back pain, had suffered shoulder pain. She could not lift her arm much higher than the horizontal position. There was pain in the front and back of the shoulder joint. In fact, even Susan's chest muscles hurt: the pectorals were chronically contracted and pulled her shoulders forward into a rounded posture.

We began the session very carefully; I was unsure of what she would be able to do. We did gentle Pelvic Tilts, Abdominal Curls, and Half Rollups using the ball. I encouraged her to go gently so that tension was not created in the neck or other parts of the body. Rolling the ball along the body helped Susan scan her body to see where she was holding discomfort or pain. Also the shape and feel of the ball aided her in visualizing the wheel image used in many of the Pilates exercises—exercises she thought she would never in a million years be able to attempt.

I wasn't so sure. Her technique was excellent. Back breathing, which she picked up easily, helped relax her and focus her mind. It was true that she felt defeated by her body and that her problems were overwhelming. However, the grace and care she took with each exercise encouraged me greatly. Her body, in spite of being racked with pain and grossly deconditioned, knew a lot! Also, the modifications we attempted did not add to her pain. At the end of the session she declared exuberantly that she had not felt better in a long time.

On the second visit I added armwork. Because of the shoulder pain we began without weights to be sure that her body stayed properly aligned. In the next session I added one-pound weights. All the time I was watching Susan like a hawk—she had more restrictions, pain, and limitations than any student I had taken on. Yet she surprised me with each session.

The wonderful thing about the ball is that it helps people sit in good posture while performing the exercises. Susan sat tall on her ball and even did gentle bouncing, which she felt was pleasant, not painful. Gentle rotation and small side bends, usually discouraged with lower back pain and disk problems, did not seem to affect her—except positively. I reminded her never to combine bouncing with rotation or twisting of the spine and gave her a series of home exercises.

The ball is known to encourage people who might not be bothered to practice their home rehabilitation exercises. The comfort, shape, and pleasant associations of the ball inspire people of all ages to workout on their own, and Susan was no exception. "The ball feels like an extension of my own body," she told me. The more she practiced the exercises on her own, the stronger her body became. She was well on her way to being able to join a basic-level group class and did so three months later.

Muscles Do Remember

Many people believe that as physical beings we have lived many lives and each has left an indelible mark. Recalling injuries dredges up painful memories. But as any bodywork practitioner will tell you, each injury tells a story: a pattern of one's physical compulsions, imbalances, and obsessions. Injury is a gift for learning—if we choose to see it in that manner. Recurring pain forces us to examine how our bodies are really working and what our true limitations and strengths are. This knowledge is crucial in rebuilding our bodies and preventing injuries from repeating themselves.

According to somatics pioneer Thomas Hanna, many pains, restrictions, and injuries are caused by the body's response to stress and trauma. Our sensory-motor systems respond to daily strains and demands with specific muscular reflexes. It is not within our control to relax these reflexes once they are triggered. Muscular contractions are involuntary and unconscious. Without proper exercise we eventually forget how to move about freely. The result is stiffness, soreness, and a restricted range of motion. Hanna calls it sensory-motor amnesia.

Many practitioners and somatic educators believe that the body can remember how to move properly again. The ill effects of sensory-motor amnesia can be reversed. Muscles do remember previous incarnations—a time before the shoulder injury, the arthritis, and the back pain.

For example, in her youth Susan had been physically active. She had developed heart and muscle strength from aerobic classes and had a dancer's grace and flexibility. I could detect this within minutes of working with her. Even though we were working with very small movements, and even if there were times she didn't believe that she could exercise again, *her body did*. Week by week we sorted through her muscle history like sifting through deposits of sediment, gently digging deeper into her muscle past, unearthing a time when mobility was free and boundless. The Pilates on the Ball exercises we did together, and those Susan did on her own, were a major part of this excavation. It was the act of movement that helped her muscles remember.

The body is a mystery; even with painstaking effort to understand it, one can be fooled. It is better not to try to self-diagnose; if you have chronic pain, or when the simple remedies presented in this book do not appear to offer relief, seek medical advice. Then take that advice and totally commit to participating in your own rebuilding program.

Pain Reduction

It is important to remember that most pain is not simply situated in one area but radiates into other parts of the body. A practitioner can help you decipher where the pain is really coming from and what is causing the problem. Is the pain the result of an imbalance between muscle groups, or a chronic holding pattern of tension in a particular part of the body? Is there something in the way you hold your body in exercise and normal activities that is contributing to the problem?

Restoration of good posture is essential to addressing pain. Poor alignment problems can be transferred directly to the fitness class or the swimming pool. Look in a mirror when performing exercises or have a few sessions with a trainer to see what the problem is and how to avoid it in the future. Ask yourself after each session if you feel better or worse. Follow Thomas Hanna's refrain: "Always move slowly, gently, and without forcing the movement."

With modest lower back pain, lie on your back with your calf muscles up on the ball. This is a safe way to let the back settle. Take care not to force down the tailbone and exaggerate the lower back curve. Breathe deeply and allow at least fifteen minutes for the body's weight to release into the mat.

If you have a mild neck strain, place your hands behind your neck and gently lift your head using your hands and not your neck muscles. Hold your head up, drop your chin, and give the back of the neck a small stretch. Carefully place the head back on the mat and repeat. The neck, shoulders, and lower back store daily tension. If your neck tension is more severe, or you have chronic pain or tension, it is best to see a doctor, physical therapist, or chiropractor.

Sitting on the ball is sometimes all you can do if you are in pain. Gentle bouncing mobilizes the spine and can release pain. Stop immediately if it adds discomfort. Use a mirror to be sure that you are not exaggerating the lower back curve into a pain-enhancing lordotic arch.

A small extension and the resistance of gravity can gently lengthen tight segments of the back. If you have worked with your ball a bit and have already mastered the Arch, try a smaller version of it called the Tabletop (both exercises are detailed in the next chapter). The Tabletop, like the Arch, can reduce compression in the lower back and create separation between pelvis and ribs while at the same time working the small back muscles. Be sure that you support the buttocks from below and use your abdominals. Both of these moves also release the neck while totally supporting it at the same time. The Arch is a very powerful stretch, and I would avoid it if you have lower back pain. If you are not warmed up or if you hold this particular stretch for too long you may feel your back tense up to protect itself from the unaccustomed feeling of space in the body. To come out of the Tabletop put the hands behind the head to lift the head, chin to chest.

Take care as you roll in and out of these recuperative positions. Afterward ask yourself what you feel. Do you feel better than before or worse?

The Role of Abdominals in Back Care

As discussed in chapter 4, it is widely believed that abdominal strength will help heal and prevent lower back pain. Pay attention to how abdominal exercises are performed. Vigorous, swift crunches work the abdominals but cause them to become short and contracted. Often these crunches are performed with too much movement; consequently the action recruits the powerful hip flexors, which may also become tight. In Pilates on the Ball we are attempting not only to strengthen the abdominals but also to lengthen them.

89

We need to be able to activate the deep transversus abdominals and not simply suck in the belly. If the abdominal muscles protrude while performing the exercises it is a sure sign that the connection has been lost. I encourage students to press a finger just below the navel to make sure that the abdominal wall is drawn in. Take care when lying on the abdomen or with the belly on the ball to be sure that the navel is lifted up and off the mat or the ball. This contraction must be held while movements are added and must not interfere with the breathing pattern. To help maintain the navel-to-spine connection and protect the small of the back, breath is directed into the rib cage and not into the abdominals.

Shoulder and Neck Problems

The first thing you must do with shoulder and neck pain is to diligently examine the ins and outs of your day to learn what is contributing to your condition. For example, a job that requires you to work frequently on one side and in one position, such as a dental hygienist or violinist, could cause problems early in life. Maybe the solution to your neck pain is to use a headset instead of crunching the phone between your shoulder and ear. Do you spend your days slumped forward over a computer with your shoulders up around your ears? Changing to an ergonomically designed kneeling chair, or using a ball for your desk chair, would greatly aid in supporting better posture at your desk.

The responsibilities of our lives cause us to move through our days "head first," causing imbalances in the body. Thomas Hanna referred to this as the "green light reflex." It is a reflex of activity and urgency that is triggered constantly by the demands of a busy lifestyle. According to Hanna, the other reflex, which we wear around our body like a cloak, is the "red light reflex," or withdrawal response. It is a protective response to fear or distressing events. This reflex triggers tension in the neck muscles and can result in a forward-projected head. It also manifests in the shoulders, causing them to lift and round forward.

Good alignment of the shoulder girdle is important. The shoulders should be down and stabilized before you do any movement. Cultivate an awareness of easing the shoulder blades down the back without forcing the latissimus dorsi down and causing lack of mobility in the arm joint. Because the head is heavy, we need to ensure that the head is aligned and not held forward on the body.

When exercising with neck and shoulder tension, leave the head on the mat when indicated. You may want to avoid using the ball during the abdominal exercises, as it adds one or two pounds of resistance that may aggravate neck pain. Take care at all times with the placement of the head on the mat as well as when sitting upright on the ball.

The Ball as Therapeutic Partner

While she was crossing the street on a green light, Eve was knocked down in the crosswalk by a car. A vertebra in her lower back was fractured, and she spent two and half weeks in the hospital numb from the waist down. Eve, a fifty-two-year-old former dancer, was a physical fitness and yoga instructor and feared that she would never teach movement again.

Most physicians approach exercise after an injury by focusing on starting rehabilitation as soon as possible. Eve's doctor was no exception. He considered the nature of the injury as well as Eve's kinesthetic awareness as a yoga teacher and believed she would be a good candidate for a slow but steady recovery. She was used to working hard as a dancer and did everything she could to contribute to her own rehabilitation.

When Eve came to my ball class she was teaching again, but her body had not recovered fully. She could not even do a small Bridge and feared that the Wheel or *Cakrasana*, the big extension of yoga, was a pose of the past. "The ball was a big surprise," she told me after her first class. "The ball stabilized me so I could try things I never thought I could do."

Eve's spine craved the dynamic extension of the arch and the exercise ball brought this extension within her reach by two and a half months. In the final class of a ten-week course she lay backward over the ball, stretching her hands in one direction and her feet in the other. She had brought her camera to class. She asked me to snap a photo of her in extension to show her doctor.

The ball has a long history of use with orthopedic patients. It is used in testing and assessing patients and then used directly by the patient to restrengthen the trunk and increase the range of motion of the trunk, legs, and arms. The ball can also save the therapist's back by taking the weight of a weak or paralyzed leg. Physical therapists and those using the ball for rehabilitation should read Beate Carrière's excellent book, *The Swiss Ball: Theory, Basic Exercises and Clinical Application*. Carrière explains that one of the many rewards of the ball is that it can be used to control the amount of weight-bearing on the hand or leg. This is beneficial in rehabilitating a shoulder or knee after injury or surgery. In a push-up, for example, the trunk is fully supported by the ball. Taking care not to lower the body past elbow level, the shoulder will not be stressed as it would in a full weight-bearing situation. With wrist problems you can control how much weight is taken on the wrist by how far you walk out on the ball. For frozen shoulder and other injuries, the ball can be used by the patient to mobilize the arm and to increase the range of movement in the shoulder without having to lift the arm.

For the same reason, the ball is an excellent therapeutic partner after knee ligament reconstruction and hip or knee replacements. Using a ball elevates the leg and allows the affected leg to rest on the ball while moving it. The patient is challenged to keep the leg aligned while moving the knee in flexion and extension. Most important, he or she is in control of the movement.

The Rebuilding Exercises

The key to injury prevention is utilizing all of the body, balancing all of its parts. The exercises in this chapter focus on core stabilization and test core strength. This is one way of revealing where there may be a muscle imbalance and setting out from there. As you work through the exercises pay close attention to which ones can be done with pain and which cannot. Some of these exercises are only to be attempted when your pain is gone and you are ready to rebuild or strengthen your healthy body. Do not push yourself too hard; only progress when you are pain-free and you have mastered the basic work. If you are in doubt about an exercise, leave it out.

This chapter presents some of the most advanced work in the entire book. Some of you, including myself, do not need to do advanced work and will never miss it in our bodies. For others, especially elite athletes and dancers, the challenge and novelty of doing advanced Pilates on the Ball will greatly enhance their performance. The advanced work often involves taking away the base of support and working with the body as a longer lever. For this reason, the farther the ball is off-center, the more resistance is added and the greater the demand for core stability. Take care to notice that the advanced work is clearly marked, so if you are a beginner you will not stumble into it by accident. Quite often a modification is shown, and you can attempt a smaller version of a more advanced exercise.

Hip Rolls

Small Hip Rolls can be done with modest lower back pain; a small sequencing movement is usually good to release the muscles in the lower back and create mobility in the spine. Take care when you return the pelvis to the mat not to exaggerate the curve in the lower back by forcing down the tailbone and making a larger space in the lower back than is beneficial. Try to feel the vertebrae move individually, separately, not in a block. Remember: the farther the ball is away from your torso, the more difficult the exercise.

Purpose To sequence through the body and create mobility in the spine.
Watchpoints • Do not overarch at the top; lift the pelvis only a couple of inches if you have lower back pain. • Connect through the inner thighs; try not to let the legs separate on the ball. • The neck should be relaxed, shoulders melting and widening.

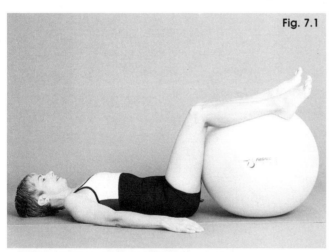

Fig. 7.1

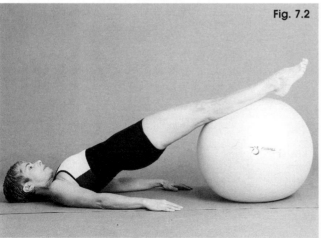

Fig. 7.2

starting position

Lie on your back with your calf muscles resting on the ball and your hands by the side of your thighs (fig. 7.1). Connect through the inner thighs. Be sure that the shoulders are sliding down away from your ears.

movement

1. Inhale to lengthen the tailbone away from the pelvis.
2. Exhale to continue to lengthen and curl the tailbone up one vertebra at a time until your body is in a straight line, shoulders in line with toes (fig. 7.2).
3. Inhale at the top.
4. Exhale to soften through the chest and sequence down one vertebra at a time.

93

Hip Rolls with Balance

Attempt this balancing movement only when your body is feeling strong and pain-free. In this exercise we are testing the core strength of the body by decreasing the solid base of support. The whole body must work together here or you may roll off the ball completely.

Purpose To strengthen the torso and test core balance.
Watchpoints • Do not overarch at the top by lifting the pelvis too high.
• Connect through the inner thighs. • Be sure your neck is relaxed.

starting position

Lie on your back with your calf muscles resting on the ball and your hands by the side of your thighs. Connect through the inner thighs. Be sure that the shoulders are sliding down away from your ears.

movement 1

1. Inhale to lengthen the tailbone away from the pelvis.
2. Exhale to continue to lengthen and curl the tailbone up one vertebra at a time until your body is in a straight line, shoulders in line with toes.
3. Hold this position, breathing normally and connecting through the buttocks, inner thighs, and abdominals.
4. Leaving elbows on the mat, slowly lift wrists and hands off the mat (fig. 7.3). Breathe naturally and hold for a few counts.
5. Exhale to soften through the chest and sequence down one vertebra at a time.

movement 2—intermediate

1. Same movement as above except this time raise the hands to the ceiling, lifting the tips of the shoulder blades off the mat (fig. 7.4) and further reducing your support from stable ground. Breathe naturally and hold for a few counts.
2. Exhale to soften through the chest and sequence down one vertebra at a time.

movement 3—advanced

1. Same movement as above except lift the head off the mat as well (fig. 7.5). Breathe naturally and hold for a few counts.
2. Exhale to soften through the chest and sequence down one vertebra at a time.

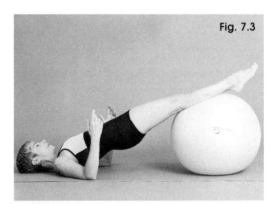

Fig. 7.3

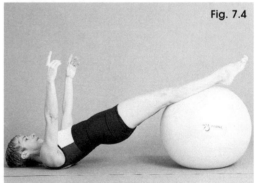

Fig. 7.4

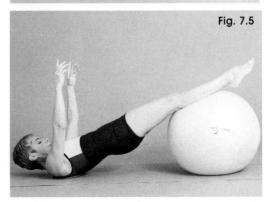

Fig. 7.5

Shoulder Bridges

Avoid this movement if you have lower back pain. In addition to strengthening the abdominals, Shoulder Bridges work the backs of the legs, the buttocks, and the hamstrings. Do not overextend the spine by lifting the pelvis too high; instead focus on a deep abdominal connection and keeping the spine in neutral. When you lift one leg off the ball you are decreasing the base of support much more than on a mat because the ball is unstable, and there is only one leg on it. Deep muscles should hold their contraction throughout, with abdominals flat and pelvis steady, while you change legs. If you have recently had knee surgery and can't fully extend the knee, keep to movement 1.

Do not rush these bridges. There is a slow breath for each movement.

Purpose To work the torso and strengthen the backs of the legs, hamstrings, and buttocks.

Watchpoints • Keep your kneecaps facing toward the ceiling throughout the movement. • Use the abdominal obliques to close the ribs so you don't overextend in the chest area. • Be sure that the buttocks are working to keep the hips up and in place. • If you cannot fully straighten the moving leg, make the motion smaller. • Keep motions small to gain control.

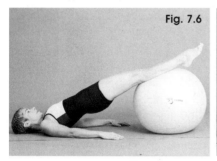

Fig. 7.6

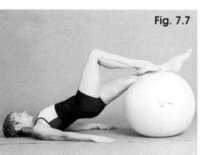

Fig. 7.7

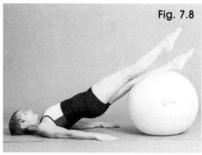

Fig. 7.8

starting position

Lie on your back with your calf muscles resting on the ball and your hands by the side of your thighs. Connect through the inner thighs. Be sure that the shoulders are sliding down away from your ears.

movement 1: preparation for shoulder bridge

1. Inhale to prepare.
2. Exhale to lift the hips using the buttock muscles (fig. 7.6).
3. Inhale to bend the right leg, bringing the toes to the left ankle (fig. 7.7).
4. Exhale to extend the right leg two inches above the ball (fig. 7.8).
5. Inhale and stay.

6. Exhale to return a straight leg to the ball. Squeeze buttocks and inner thighs and remain in place.
7. Inhale to bend left leg and bring toe to right ankle.
8. Exhale to extend left leg two inches above the ball.
9. Inhale stay.
10. Exhale to return a straight leg to the ball and roll hips down to the mat.
11. Repeat twice on each side.

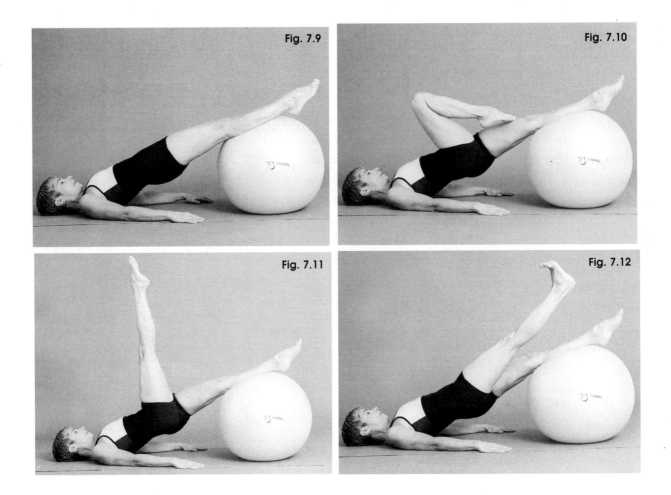

Fig. 7.9 Fig. 7.10 Fig. 7.11 Fig. 7.12

movement 2: full shoulder bridge—advanced

1. Inhale to prepare.

2. Exhale to lift the hips using the buttock muscles (fig. 7.9).

3. Inhale to bend the right leg, bringing the toes to the side of the left knee (fig. 7.10).

4. Exhale to extend the right leg straight in the air, toes pointed, leg as straight as possible (fig. 7.11).

5. Inhale to flex the foot, pushing out with the heel as you lower the right leg (fig. 7.12).

6. Exhale to lift the right leg, keeping the leg straight and pointing the foot.

7. Inhale to flex the foot and reach the heel away from you as you lower the right leg.

8. Exhale to lift the right leg, pointing the foot.

9. Repeat the lowering and lifting of the leg three times and then gently squeeze the buttocks before switching to the other side. Repeat twice on both sides.

Hip Lift

You will feel this exercise in the backs of the legs and in the hamstrings and calf muscles. If you have had knee surgery or lower back pain, perform only movement 1. Also be aware of the luxurious, air-filled quality of the ball as it rubs the bottoms of the feet and the heels.

Purpose To tone and strengthen the buttocks and hamstrings.

Watchpoint • Try to keep tension out of other parts of the body.

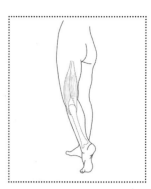

anatomy on the ball: hamstrings

Short hamstrings are known to hamper mobility in the body; they cause not only bad posture but lower back pain. This is due to the attachment points of this group of three muscles to the body.

The hamstring muscles originate on the sitz bones at the bottom of the pelvis and span across the back of the legs to attach on the inside and the outside of the back of the knee near the top of the calf muscle. Pass your hand down the body where these long muscles are and think of the implications of shortness on the rest of the body, especially the pelvis. Hamstring stretches are shown in the next chapter.

starting position

Lie on your back with the bottoms of your feet on the ball, knees bent, hands beside your thighs and slightly extended, shoulders down and relaxed (fig. 7.13).

movement 1: without hip lift

1. Keeping your pelvis on the mat, inhale to roll the ball out using the bottoms of the feet (fig. 7.14).
2. Exhale to pull the ball back in with the heels.
3. Inhale out.
4. Exhale in.
5. Roll the ball in and out six to eight times.

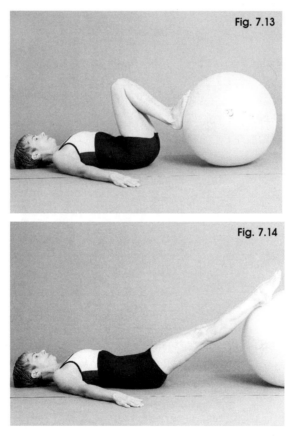

Fig. 7.13

Fig. 7.14

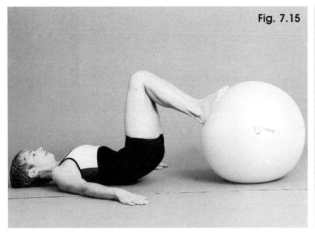

Fig. 7.15

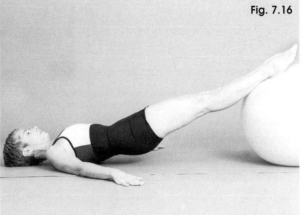

Fig. 7.16

movement 2: hip lift—intermediate

1. Place your feet on the ball. Inhale to prepare.
2. Exhale to squeeze the buttocks and lift the pelvis two or three inches, staying in neutral pelvis (fig. 7.15).

3. Inhale to roll the ball out (fig. 7.16) and exhale to pull the ball back in.
4. Repeat six to eight times.

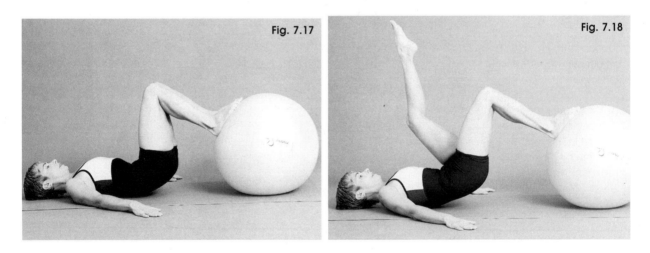

Fig. 7.17

Fig. 7.18

movement 3: one leg hip lift—advanced

1. Inhale to prepare.
2. Exhale to squeeze the buttocks and lift the pelvis two or three inches (fig. 7.17).

3. Inhale to lift the left leg in the air (fig. 7.18).
4. Exhale and stay.
5. Inhale to roll the ball out. Exhale to pull the ball in.
6. Repeat five times. Lower your pelvis to the mat before changing to the right leg.

Bend and Stretch

The abdominals work hard in this exercise. On the exhale sink them into the back of the spine as you extend the legs. If you have lower back pain, keep the legs very high in the air and perform only movement 1.

Purpose To tone the abdominals, legs, hip adductor muscles, and inner thighs.

Watchpoints • Try not to let the body sink between the shoulders.

• Maintain stability in the abdominals.

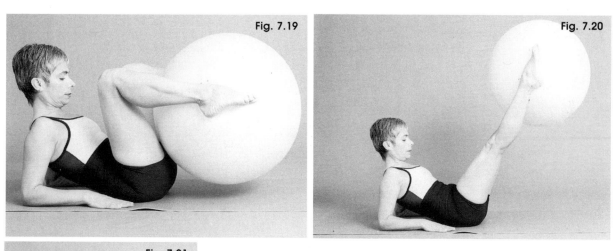

Fig. 7.19

Fig. 7.20

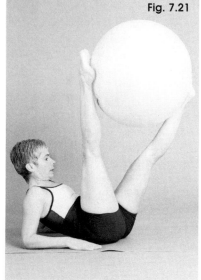

Fig. 7.21

starting position

1. Lie on your back with knees bent. Pick up the ball between your ankles and squeeze. Bend the knees in.
2. Sit up and rest the upper body on your elbows (fig. 7.19).

movement 1: bend and stretch

1. Inhale to prepare.
2. Exhale to extend the legs 45 degrees or higher from the floor (fig. 7.20).
3. Inhale to draw the ball into you and exhale to extend the legs.
4. Perform this exercise six to eight times.

movement 2: ball twist—intermediate

1. Extend legs 45 degrees or higher from the floor.
2. Keeping the legs straight, swivel the ball from side to side (fig. 7.21) and breathe naturally.

On the Side

The sidework isolates the muscles of the leg and gives us the opportunity to work the front and the back of the body together. The abdominals are critical here for keeping the torso very stable while you are moving your legs. You do not need to lift the ball higher than two inches; if you feel any discomfort in the side of the waist then you are probably working the ball too high. If you have lower back pain focus on gently squeezing the ball between the feet and do not lift.

Purpose To strengthen the inner and outer thighs and the buttocks. To tone the inner thighs as you squeeze the ball.

Watchpoints • Be careful not to take the ball behind the body. • Use a small piece of foam if your hips are bony and you find it uncomfortable to lie on your side. • Think of stretching the ball away from you rather than bringing the legs up high. • Maintain abdominal connection throughout.

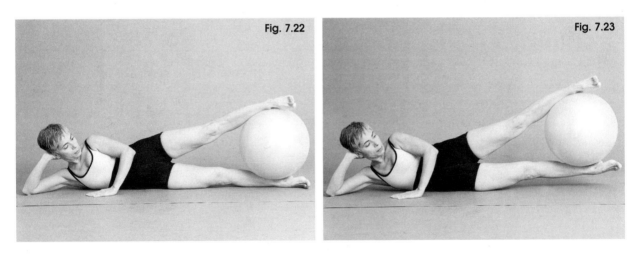

Fig. 7.22   Fig. 7.23

starting position

1. Lie on your side, one hipbone on top of the other, with the ball between your ankles.
2. One hand can rest behind your head, elbows folded (fig. 7.22), or relax the head down on the mat. Place the other hand on the mat to retain balance.

movement

1. Inhale to lengthen the heels as far away from the pelvis as possible, and squeeze the ball.
2. Exhale to lift the ball two or three inches (fig. 7.23).
3. Inhale to lower the ball. Exhale to lift.
4. Repeat five times on both sides.

Ball Balance

Everything in the Pilates Method is done with precision, focus, and concentration, and this move puts all these principles to the test. Concentrate and have patience; your legs may shake as you try to find the moment of calm in the middle of this tricky balance. If there is tightness in the hips or hamstrings, getting the ball in place will be challenging, even impossible for some. Instead, try the movement against the wall.

Purpose To challenge your sense of balance and work the back of the legs and abdominals.

Watchpoints • Do not rush in or out of the balance. • Be sure that your feet are sitz-bone distance apart.

starting position

Lie on your back with the ball in your hands. Bend the knees into your chest and slowly attempt to rest the ball on the soles, not the sides, of your feet. Feet should be sitz-bone-distance apart (fig. 7.24).

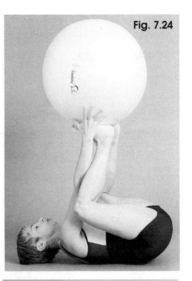

Fig. 7.24

movement 1

1. Slowly straighten your legs, keeping the ball balanced on the bottoms of your feet (fig. 7.25).
2. Breathe naturally.
3. When the legs are completely straight, hold the balance for as long as you like.
4. Slowly bend the legs, eventually taking the ball into your hands.

movement 2

1. Scoot your buttocks to four to six inches away from a wall.
2. Place the ball against the wall and slowly roll it up the wall with your feet. Balance the ball as much as you can on the soles, not the sides, of your feet. Your feet should be sitz-bone distance apart.
3. Stay in this position for a few moments, taking some deep breaths.

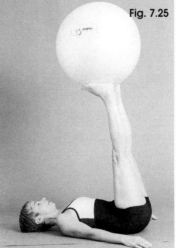

Fig. 7.25

101

The Push-up

In this exercise the entire body, not just the arms or shoulders, works as a strong unit. With the legs resting on the ball there is time and support for pulling the abdominals up, checking hand-shoulder alignment, and adjusting head placement and lower body alignment. Movement 1 is fine to use with modest lower back pain but be doubly sure that the abdominals are engaged so that the lower back is protected. Whatever you do, do not slump down and sink in the middle. By far the biggest weakness people have with the Push-up is in the gluteals, the muscles of the buttocks. They do not think about the fact that the buttocks and inner thighs need to squeeze together.

You do not have to lower the body very far to be effective; start with a very small bend and stretch of the arms. As in most ball exercises the farther the ball is away from the torso the more difficult the move.

Purpose To work the chest and shoulder muscles and the entire torso.
Watchpoints • In order to maintain good stability in the shoulder girdle you may not want to lower the body too far. • Keep your shoulder blades open across the back and not pinching together as you perform the Push-up. • Do not let your elbows jar into place when you straighten the arms. • Avoid swayback. Keep the abdominals connected. • Squeeze the inner thighs and buttocks. • Do not let the head drop: keep it in line with the spine.

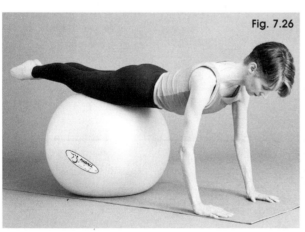

Fig. 7.26

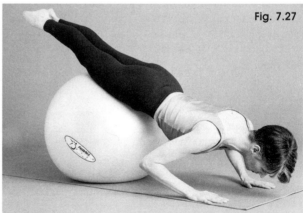

Fig. 7.27

starting position
Kneel in front of the ball.

movement 1—basic

102

1. Place hands palm-down on the floor. Walk out, keeping hands just wider than the shoulders until the ball is right in front of the knees (on the thighs). Fingertips should be parallel to the body (fig. 7.26).
2. Inhale to bend the arms (fig. 7.27). Keep the movement small at first.
3. Exhale to straighten the arms.
4. Repeat six to eight times.

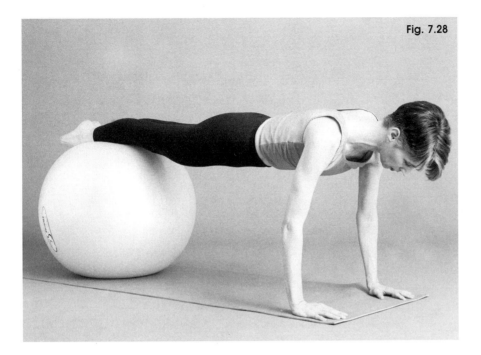

Fig. 7.28

movement 2—intermediate

1. Begin this movement in the same way as movement 1, except walk out until the ball is on the other side of the knees (at the top of the shins).
2. Inhale to bend the arms.
3. Exhale to straighten the arms.
4. Repeat six to eight times.

movement 3: advanced push-up

1. Begin this movement in the same way as movement 1, except walk out until the ball is on the ankles (fig. 7.28).
2. Inhale to bend the arms.
3. Exhale to straighten the arms.
4. Repeat six to eight times.
5. To further intensify the move try lifting one leg two inches from the ball, then attempt a small push-up. Keep both legs very straight.

The Pike

The Pike is an advanced move intended to challenge an already strong body. Movements 1 and 2 are supreme abdominal exercises that work the upper body. Try to keep the legs absolutely straight and connected as you attempt to lift the pelvis with the abdominals. Be sure that the area around you is clear in case you lose your balance.

Purpose To strengthen the arms and abdominals.
Watchpoints • The legs must remain very straight during this advanced move. • Imagine that you are suspended from the abdominals by a strong spring attached to the ceiling. • Keep the body steady while in the Pike, shoulders down and in place.

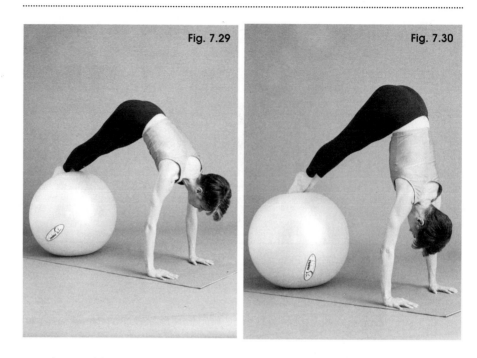

Fig. 7.29   Fig. 7.30

starting position

Place your hands palm-down on the floor. Walk out keeping the hands just wider than shoulder-distance apart until the ball is on the shins. Hands should be in place on the floor shoulder-distance apart or wider. Fingertips are parallel to the body.

movement 1—intermediate

1. Keeping your legs very straight, inhale to prepare.
2. Exhale to lift the pelvis a few inches using the abdominals (fig. 7.29).
3. Inhale to the plank position.
4. Exhale to lift the pelvis.
5. Repeat the movement three to five times.

movement 2—advanced

1. Roll the ball down to the shins or ankles. Be sure that the entire torso is in place: buttocks and inner thighs connected, head aligned on spine and not dropped. Inhale to prepare.
2. Exhale to lift the pelvis as high as possible. Use your abdominals. Do not let the legs bend (fig. 7.30).
3. Inhale to lower to the plank position.
4. Exhale to lift into a Pike. Go as high as you can without losing control.
5. Hold the Pike for a few counts, breathing naturally.
6. Repeat this movement three to five times.

You worked very hard in this section and are now in for a luxurious treat. In the next chapter you will learn how to use the ball to stretch and elongate the body safely. Many studies reveal the power of stretching for preventing injury and reviving tight, tired muscles. The ball is one of the most unique and pleasurable aids for stretching available. The spherical shape of the ball and its relaxing, air-filled support will inspire you, as it has so many others, to make stretching an everyday activity.

8

The Simplest of Pleasures: Stretching

Jeff's Story

When Jeff first arrived at a Pilates on the Ball group class he wondered if he was in the right place. For him, that was. He knew he had the correct address. He entered a spacious room, sparse of furniture except for sixteen large pearl-white Fitballs. Wearing gray track pants and a T-shirt, and with feet that were bare for the first time in a very long time, he quietly took a ball and made a place for himself near the back corner of the room.

Jeff was fifty, a former rower who kept his physique up as best he could with aerobic workouts, weight rooms, and the occasional skiing trip. But as much as he was maintaining some of his former strength, he could feel his body getting tighter. Short muscles, he knew, would eventually change joint position, limit range of motion, and even affect the length of his stride as he aged. He knew that a good stretching routine was prevention against the stiffness and dreadful morning achiness that he often felt, but found the stretches he performed at his gym neither beneficial nor pleasurable. In fact, they were downright boring. The truth was he often rushed through his stretches as if they were a series of chores—forcing his muscles to "relax" and commanding his body to release. He could hardly hold a single stretch for five seconds, never mind the 40 to 60 seconds suggested by the stretching charts.

Jeff had been interested in exercise balls ever since he had seen on television that they were used with astonishing results by Olympic coaches. He was intrigued that professional athletes were using what looked like oversized beachballs for strengthening and stretching. That was when he began to make inquiries.

One of the first things Jeff discovered in his Pilates on the Ball class was that the lengthening or opening of the muscle is as important as the shortening or contraction of the muscle. This was almost the opposite of most weight-lifting sessions where he had watched men and women heave a weight into place and then lower it as if the latter movement were just an afterthought. He was also impressed that flexibility and strength-building components were often included in the same ball exercise. Through this he was getting a lot more stretching in than he realized.

Near the end of the class we did some muscle-specific stretches. Jeff dreaded this part, fearing the stretches would hurt and that he would be discouraged by his tightness. Instead, he was amazed at how the ball comfortably but firmly supported his body. Assisted by gravity, and breath, he was able to finally get his muscles to surrender. Later he told me how he loved the way he could control the amount of stretch. By making a small adjustment in the position of the ball he would loosen the tension in the hip or hamstring and then, after a few seconds of release, roll the ball a fraction of an inch deeper into the stretch. Between classes he worked at home on stretching with his ball and after a few weeks felt his body open in a way he never dreamed possible. His morning achiness subsided.

The Benefits of Stretching

The benefits of stretching are as great for the ordinary person as they are for the athlete. In Dr. Steven D. Stark's excellent book on stretching, *The Stark Reality of Stretching*, the anatomical reasons for stretching, especially stretching the lower extremities, are clearly spelled out. Muscles shorten over time with activities as gentle as sitting or as vigorous as speed skating. It is crucial to elongate shortened muscles back to their best resting position, as tight muscles influence the movement of the lower back and pelvis and can cause pain, especially if tightness is asymmetrical. Moreover, muscle shortening affects the joints and ligaments around the muscle. This can eventually lead to recurring injuries, poor posture, and pain. What we are aiming for when we stretch is muscular balance and length in all the muscle groups. In addition, regular stretching will promote circulation, increase range of motion, and make the body feel more relaxed.

In addition to benefiting the general public, Dr. Stark is convinced that stretching assists athletes greatly. If athletes do not stretch faithfully prior to athletic performance, they will never achieve their full potential in sports. Muscles have the most power when the individual muscle fibers are at their

did you hug your ball today?

Touch is the first sense to develop inside the womb. The unique air-filled quality of the ball and its spherical shape help to reawaken a sense of touch and put us back into contact with our bodies.

In some cultures tactile awareness is as important as visual perception. As you bounce, glide, suspend, and explore with your ball be aware of how the sphere feels against your body. "The first sense to ignite, touch is often the last to burn out," writes Frederich Sachs, "long after our eyes betray us, our hands remain faithful to the world."

longest length during contraction. Many athletes have too much strength that is not balanced by enough or appropriate stretches. Strength and muscle mass are usually concurrent with tightness. Athletes can be very set in their ways when it comes to stretching. Often the strongest hockey players or weightlifters I have worked with have the tightest bodies and are less powerfully agile than their teammates who have taken dance or stretch classes. Without the proper stretching program in place athletes are very vulnerable to injury and may suffer chronically with pain to the knees, hips, and back.

Even if we are not athletes, stretching must become second nature. Like a cat that constantly stretches its limbs and flexes its spine, we must stretch to ease the backbone, relax our muscles, and prevent problems as we age. Joseph Pilates was said to have studied the movements of animals; he knew that symmetry and lengthening of muscles was as important in body maintenance as developing pure strength. One of the wonderful aspects of his method is how so many of the exercises have stretching and strengthening components integrated into the same exercise.

When it comes to a tool for stretching, the ball has no equal. Ball stretches are full and luxurious. Using the tug of gravity to maximum benefit, the sleek sphere of the ball opens the body, helps you focus on the part of the body you are stretching, and allows you to get in touch with where you are holding strain. In addition, the air-filled quality of the ball safely supports and relaxes the body so that the muscles involved can release and elongate rather than tense up involuntarily while trying to hold the body upright.

Ball stretches are not about how far you can go. Nor are they about forcing the body to recapture a position you so easily gained in youth. Ball stretches are solitary, pleasurable, and relaxing, and totally adjustable to the individual. Stretching is also a great stress buster: it relaxes your mind as it tunes your body's structural and muscular imbalances.

The Ins and Outs of Safe Stretches

The ball will help you stretch safely and effectively even if all you do are the stretches shown in this chapter. However, whether you are an athlete about to participate in a competitive event or a beginner trying out a ball stretch for the first time, it is important that you warm up before you stretch. Stretching should never be used to warm up the body. The Pilates on the Ball matwork, armwork, or footwork is a great way to heat the muscles, but if you are not beginning with those exercises be sure to take a ten-minute walk or do some gentle aerobic moves to warm the body. Gentle bouncing on the ball, adding arm movements, will also work to get the blood flowing into the muscles. Stretching when cold or stretching the wrong way can contribute to existing problems and even rupture or strain muscle fibers, ligaments, and joints.

The key to effective stretching is to be very present in the stretch and aware of what muscles are being stretched. Start with easy stretches at the point where you feel a mild tension. Stay comfortable in your stretch. Each stretch is a prayer to your body: do not force or judge. Use the breath to aid you. Hold each stretch for at least 30 seconds if possible. If you jerk the body into a severe position a protective mechanism will snap into place and tell your body to tense up in order to protect itself. That is why we are slowly and gently easing the body into the stretch a fraction of an inch at a time. The sensation of mild tension should remain constant and not suddenly become intense. Take care to keep the tension out of other parts of the body.

The following basic stretches are safe and effective, because if done properly the body is totally supported in the stretch and the muscles are not involuntarily struggling to stabilize the body against gravity. These basic stretches isolate one major muscle or muscle group. Dr. Stark maintains that single muscle stretches are the safest stretches you can do, and my basic ball stretches are selected with the mechanism of stretching in mind. In addition, these basic stretches are designed not to put the lower back in a damaging position where stress on the pelvic, spinal ligaments, or sciatic nerve could occur. Near the end of the chapter are a few advanced stretches that may stretch more than one muscle group or part of the body that must work to stabilize or keep the body upright. This level of stretch is for the very fit and flexible.

The Stretching Exercises

The following Pilates on the Ball stretches have your name on them. But before you glide into them be aware of a few time-tested precautions.

- Do not force the stretch.

- Never bounce into the stretch or jerk out of it.

- Try to keep tension out of other parts of the body.

- Be aware of your alignment during the stretch.

- There is no competition. Adjust each stretch to suit *your* body. Understretching is better than overstretching.

- Use the exhale to ease a fraction of an inch deeper into the stretch.

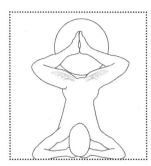

anatomy on the ball: the groin muscles

Adduction of the hip— movement of the hip toward the body in the frontal plane—is the primary function of the groin muscles. These muscles, located in the inner thighs, help to stabilize the femur and connect it to the pelvis. The groin muscles are frequently torn if not warmed up or stretched properly.

Frog Stretch

The following exercise is a comfortable, relaxing stretch that is best performed in bare feet so that the feet will not slip on the ball. The mat supports the back and there is no stress on the ligaments in the lower back or the pelvis. You are trying to stretch the inner thighs, or adductors. If these muscles are not regularly stretched they pull on the pelvis and lower back. For some people even the feet and ankle muscles will feel a stretch while in the Frog.

Purpose To stretch the inner thighs.

Watchpoints • You should feel tension in the center of the groin muscle, not high up in the groin (in the tendon). • Hold the stretch as long as it is comfortable.

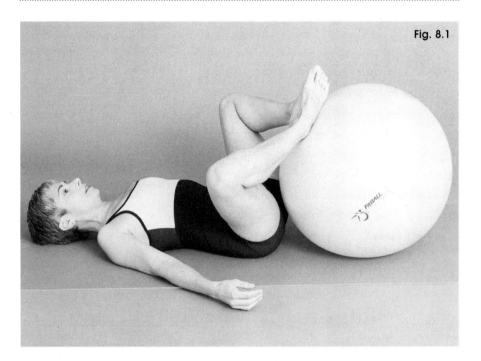

Fig. 8.1

starting position

Lie on your back with the soles of the feet together and resting on the ball. Let the knees gently open to the side in a frog-leg shape (fig. 8.1).

movement

1. Rest the hands on the inner thighs but do not force down the knees.
2. Relax. Allow gravity to ease open the inner thighs.
3. Over time you can gently ease the feet, a fraction of an inch at a time, closer to the groin area.
4. Stay in this stretch for as long as you like.

Hamstring Stretch

There are three muscles that run down the back of the thigh that make up the hamstrings. These muscles extend from the sitz bones to the inside and outside of the knee. The hamstring muscles do not stretch behind the knee; thus you should not feel this stretch in the back of the knee. If you feel pressure on the back of the knee, keep the knee slightly bent. Tight hamstrings cause poor posture and lower back pain and problems.

Purpose To stretch the hamstrings.

Watchpoints • In all three movements the tailbone should remain on the mat. • In movements 1 and 2 be aware of the neck as you stretch. Try not to arch the back and shorten the neck. Drop the chin gently as if you have a tennis ball at the throat, or place a flat pillow under the head. • In movement 3 be aware that attempting to grab the toes or dorsiflex the foot makes the stretch more intense because it involves the calf muscle as well.

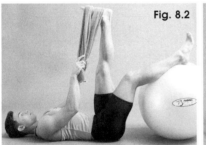
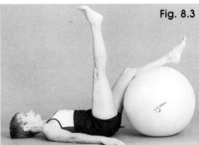
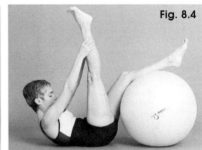

Fig. 8.2   *Fig. 8.3*   *Fig. 8.4*

starting position
Lie on your back with the back of both calves resting on the ball.

movement 1: with towel or scarf
1. Sling a towel across the arch of the left foot. Keeping the tailbone anchored on the mat, slowly straighten the left leg into the air (fig. 8.2).
2. Hold for 30 to 50 seconds. Breathe naturally.
3. Return the leg to the ball and switch sides.

movement 2: without towel
1. Lift one leg off the ball keeping the leg as straight as possible. The back of the knee can be soft. Try to keep the tailbone on the mat (fig. 8.3).
2. Hold for 5 to 20 seconds. Breathe naturally.
3. Lower the leg to the ball and switch sides.

movement 3—intermediate
1. Place both hands at the back of the thigh.
2. Inhale to prepare.
3. Exhale to slowly walk your hands up the back of the leg (fig. 8.4).
4. Inhale at the top, reaching the hand toward the toes without letting the shoulders come up.
5. Exhale to walk down the back of the leg.
6. Repeat three times on each leg.

Hip Stretch

You can move directly from the Hamstring Stretch into the Hip Stretch. The hip rotators are six small muscles that cross the back of the pelvis and are responsible for turning the thigh outward. The gluteus maximus is the large buttocks muscle. The ball is a great aid to this traditional stretch because you don't need to use the hands to pull the leg closer to the body.

Purpose To stretch the large gluteus maximus and the external hip rotators.
Watchpoints • Keep the upper body and head on the mat. • Rest the back of the pelvis evenly on the mat.

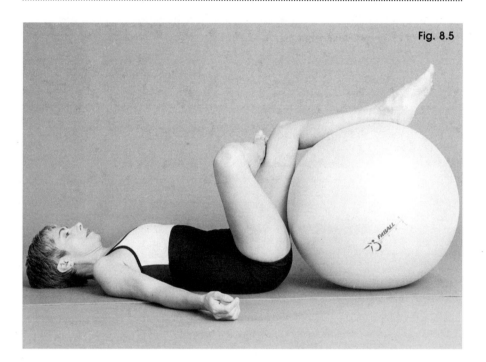

Fig. 8.5

starting position

Lie on your back with the backs of both legs resting on the ball.

movement

1. Allow the left foot to roll the ball straight out away from the body.
2. Cross the right foot over the left thigh. There should be no tension in the hip muscles.

3. Press the left heel on the ball, bend the left knee, and slowly pull the ball toward the body, keeping the right knee open (fig. 8.5). Stop when you feel a tension in the deep hip muscles and the back of the right buttock.
4. Roll the ball back out to release tension and then slowly ease it back in.
5. Do three stretches on each side. Hold for 30 to 60 seconds each.

Neck Stretch

While you are lying on the mat, stretch out the back of the neck. This is a place where many people hold a great deal of tension. Don't forget to breathe deeply during this and all the other stretches.

Purpose To stretch the upper spine and neck.

Watchpoint • Do not overstretch the neck area.

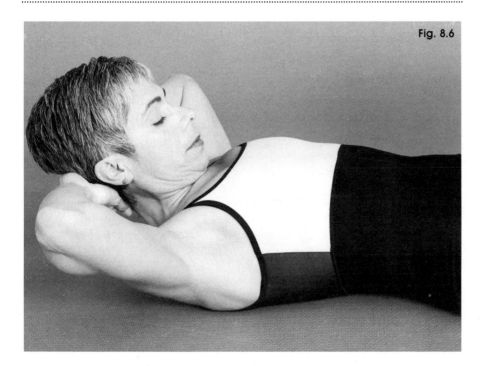

Fig. 8.6

starting position

1. Lie on your back with the back of both calves resting on the ball. Gently clasp your hands behind the head and rest them on the mat.
2. Open arms wide and feel an opening in the shoulder blades.

movement 1

1. On the exhale, and without coming up too high, slowly pull the head forward using the arm muscles (fig. 8.6). Hold for 5 to 8 seconds and then relax the head on the mat.
2. Repeat three to five times.

movement 2

1. Gently pull the head toward the right knee, without moving the knee toward the head. Hold for 6 seconds and relax head back on mat. Then pull your head toward the left knee.
2. Repeat twice on each side.

movement 3

Without lifting the head off the mat, roll the chin easily from one shoulder to the other.

The Shell

Avoid the Shell if you have knee problems. Movement 2 will isolate one arm and then the other. Avoid movement 3 if you are prone to motion sickness or if you have lower back pain. As you do the Shell practice sending the breath into the back of the rib cage. If necessary place a cushion under the ankles or between the buttocks and knees to get comfortable.

Purpose To stretch the lower and upper back, the shoulders, and the "lats," the latissimus dorsi muscle.

Watchpoint • Don't strain. If the stretch becomes too intense in the upper arms, let go of the ball and relax the hands and arms in front of you on the mat.

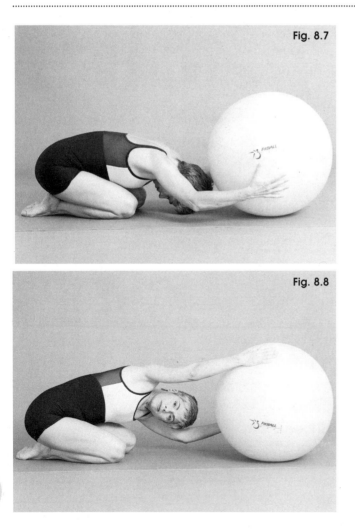

Fig. 8.7

Fig. 8.8

starting position
Kneel in front of your ball.

movement 1
1. Slowly roll the ball away from you as you sink down so that the back of the thighs come close to the buttocks. Keep your hands on the side of the ball if possible. Release your head between your arms (fig. 8.7).
2. Hold this position until it is no longer comfortable.

movement 2
1. Stretch one arm at a time by leaving one hand on the ball and the other hand on the mat in front of you.
2. Roll the ball easily from side to side to intensify the stretch.
3. Repeat twice with each arm.

movement 3: while rocking
Keeping both hands on the side of the ball, roll the ball from side to side, rotating the body and lifting the upper body to look under the arm (fig. 8.8).

114

Side Stretches

From the Shell, roll the ball to the side of the body to get into position for Side Stretches. This exercise is both a breathing exercise and a stretch. Remember on the inhale to send the breath into the side of the back rib cage. If you have knee problems push the weight onto the extended leg to get the weight off the knee. If you feel any strain in the neck hold the back of the head with your hand.

Purpose To stretch the side of the body.

Watchpoints • Take care with all three Side Stretches, especially movement 3 if you have lower back pain. • In movement 3 only go as far as is comfortable for you. Support the back of the neck with your hand if necessary. • Do not move too quickly between the three movements; very occasionally motion sickness occurs.

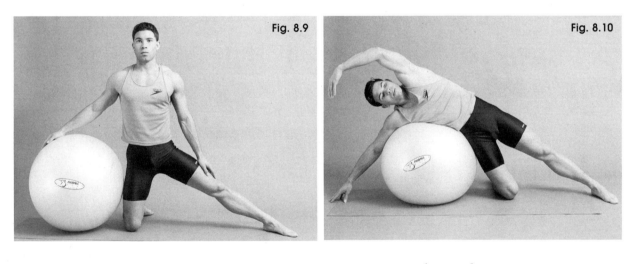

Fig. 8.9

Fig. 8.10

starting position

Kneel upright beside the ball. The ball is on your right side and the left leg is stretched out to the side (fig. 8.9). Keep the ball as close to the side of your body as possible.

movement 1: side stretch

1. Inhale to prepare and exhale to gently shift your weight to the right so that the side of the body is totally supported by the ball. Stretch the left arm over the left ear and relax the neck (fig. 8.10).
2. Take a few full, easy breaths.

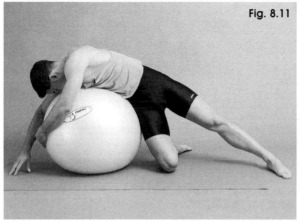

Fig. 8.11

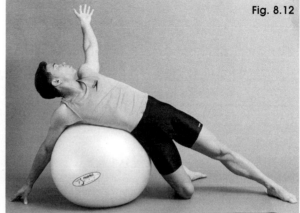

Fig. 8.12

movement 2: forward stretch

1. Inhale and exhale to drop the chest and the face onto the ball. You may want to cup the ball with the left arm (fig. 8.11).
2. Take a few breaths. The back of the neck should be totally relaxed.

movement 3: chest to ceiling

1. Inhale and exhale to lift the chest off the ball, go through the Side Stretch position, and open the chest to the ceiling (fig. 8.12).
2. Take a few breaths and then repeat movements 1, 2, and 3.
3. Switch sides by rolling the ball in front of you.

Psoas Stretch

The following exercise is an excellent stretch for hip flexibility because it stretches the powerful hip flexor muscles that lift the legs to the trunk. Take the weight onto the ball but try not to collapse over the ball.

Purpose To stretch the psoas and iliacus muscles in front of the hip.
Watchpoint • Do not position your knee forward of your ankle.

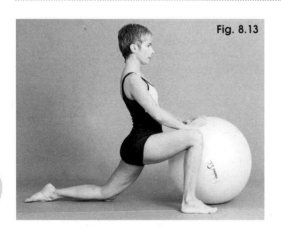

Fig. 8.13

starting position

Kneel in front of the ball. Place your hands on the top of the ball.

movement 1—basic

1. Bring the right foot forward and extend the left foot out behind you, knee resting on mat.
2. Allow the ball to roll forward to create a gentle stretch in front of the left hip. Be sure that the knee of the forward leg is directly over the ankle (fig. 8.13).
3. Hold for 20 to 30 seconds, using the ball for balance. Roll the ball back to you and switch sides to stretch both legs.

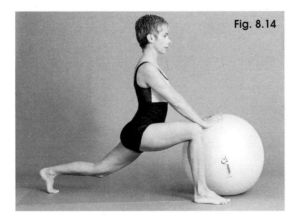

Fig. 8.14

movement 2— intermediate

1. Position yourself as in movement 1.
2. Curl the toes of the back leg and straighten and lift the knee (fig. 8.14). Hold for 20 to 30 seconds.
3. Roll the ball back to you and switch sides.

Shoulder Stretches

The space between the shoulder blades and upper arms is an area of extreme tension. Sit on your ball to do these stretches, but know that these stretches can be done any time that your body craves a deep, rejuvenating stretch.

Purpose To stretch the arms, shoulders, and upper back.
Watchpoints • Keep the breath slow and deep. • Keep the stretches comfortable, not painful.

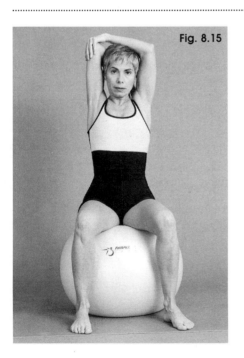

Fig. 8.15

starting position

Sit tall on the ball, feet parallel and shoulder-distance apart.

movement 1: shoulder shrug

1. Lift the top of your shoulders toward your ears. Hold for 5 seconds and drop.
2. Repeat three times.

movement 2: arms overhead

1. Lift your arms overhead and hold the elbow of one arm with the hand of the other arm (fig. 8.15).
2. Gently pull the elbow to the side. Hold for 10 to 20 seconds.
3. Stretch both sides.

117

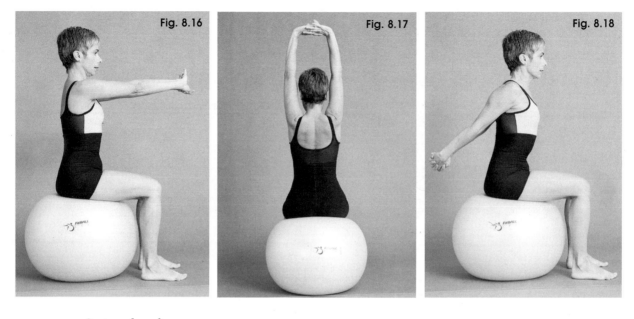

Fig. 8.16　　Fig. 8.17　　Fig. 8.18

movement 3: interlaced fingers

1. Cross your fingers and lift your arms in front of your body, palms facing outward (fig. 8.16).

2. Cross your fingers and lift your arms above your head, palms facing upward (fig. 8.17).

3. Cross your fingers and stretch your arms behind your body, palms facing each other (fig. 8.18).
4. Hold each stretch for 30 seconds.

The Arch

We spend too much of our time hunched over computers and steering wheels. Our spines, and our hearts, have forgotten how to do the carefree backbend of a child. Nothing will make you feel as refreshed and energized as the supported Arch. The abdominals are stretched, rib muscles are strengthened and opened, and internal organs are open and free. The ball gives you a stretch in the thoracic, or upper back, region, not just the flexible lower back. Let the fingers touch the floor or a chair to help you keep your balance.

The Arch is quite advanced, but you can start with a smaller version, the Tabletop, that will give you many of the same benefits. In the Tabletop the small back muscles work to keep you upright. In the Arch these muscles both contract and stretch. To come out of the Arch or the Tabletop put your hands behind your head and immediately lift the head, chin to chest.

Purpose To stretch the spine and torso. Movement 2 is also a quad or thigh stretch.

Watchpoints • Be sure that you are very warm before attempting movements 1 to 3. • The hips stay lifted in the Quad Stretch. • The neck must not be overextended; the ball must support it at all times. • Be sure that long hair does not get stuck under the ball. • Moving too quickly into the Arch can bring on motion sickness.

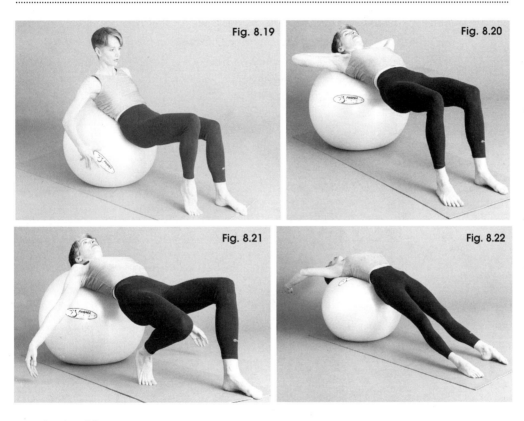

Fig. 8.19 Fig. 8.20 Fig. 8.21 Fig. 8.22

starting position
Sit on the center of your ball.

movement 1: the tabletop

1. Slowly walk your feet out in front of you. The ball will roll under you (fig. 8.19). Walk the feet out until the back of the neck and head are totally supported by the ball.
2. Gently lift the buttocks to keep the hips in line with the knees and shoulders (fig. 8.20).
3. Open the arms to a T shape to the side. Stay here and breathe for a few counts.

movement 2: with quad stretch—intermediate

1. Get into the Tabletop with the head and back of neck totally supported by the ball.

2. Gently lift the buttocks to keep hips in line with the knees and shoulders. Touch fingers to the ground to aid in balance.
3. Move one foot close to the ball. Keep the hip and heel lifted and allow the knee to drop (fig. 8.21). Hold for 20 seconds.
4. Switch legs and repeat.

movement 3: the arch—intermediate

1. For a more dynamic stretch take the arms overhead and push into the feet to arch the body over the ball (fig. 8.22).
2. Add slow, full, graceful arm circles in one direction and then the other.
3. Try peeling off an imaginary sweater.

119

The Squat

Squatting is easier on the body than standing and is encouraged in many cultures as a position of relaxation or work. The Squat is excellent for good posture; it automatically puts the body in good alignment and takes strain off the lower back. Try coming out of the Arch and sinking directly into the Squat.

Purpose To release the back and stretch hips, deep groin, ankles, and Achilles tendons. Holding the Squat will strengthen ankles and feet.
Watchpoints • Exercise caution if you have knee problems. • Knees should be aligned with toes but not jutting over toes. Move your feet out if need be.

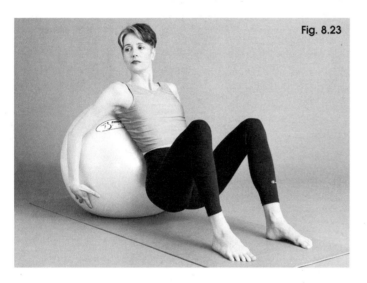

Fig. 8.23

starting position
Sit on the center of your ball.

movement
1. Walk your feet out and then bend the hips and knees and sink down. Feet are shoulder-distance apart, flat, and pointed forward, heels down. Make sure the weight is equally distributed on both feet. Your buttocks will be two or three inches off the ground (fig. 8.23).
2. Rock up and down, if desired, to give the back a massage.
3. Breathe deeply into the belly and the pelvis and hold the Squat as long as you can.

Many of the ball stretches take you back to poses that you accomplished effortlessly as children. The ball brings these positions within the reach of almost everyone. In the next chapter you will learn about bouncing on the ball and its benefits. Bouncing with balls is reminiscent of most cultures' childhood games, played either in groups or alone. Easy and safe cardiovascular exercises transferred to the ball are an effective remedy to stress and fatigue. They also enhance the fitness of the heart and lungs.

9

Stress Management and Cardiovascular Exercises

Roseanne's Story

"It's amazing I am even standing before you," Roseanne told me, brushing a honey-colored strand of hair back from her gray eyes. "This time last year I couldn't even run a comb through my hair, never mind get out of bed."

Roseanne and I were both in intensive training to become certified Pilates teachers. She had flown to Toronto from the midwestern states to do her certification with Moira Stott. I had emptied my life of all other obligations to do the same. Roseanne and I hung out a bit together. We drilled each other on anatomy and worked out together on the wonderful Pilates equipment. We also shared our stories.

Roseanne was lightly tanned and blond. She had the sort of natural good looks that made people's heads turn. She also had one of the most muscular bodies I had seen on a woman. It was an impressively sculptured body—not with the long, lean muscles associated with Pilates, but with the well-defined and bulky muscle only acquired from hours and hours of specialized training with heavy weights. Who would have guessed that fibromyalgia could have struck her body so totally?

She described the symptoms: "At first it was like having a severe bout of achy flu that went on for months. I couldn't sleep. My bones and joints were so stiff and tender that neck and shoulder pain kept me awake at night. I

121

ignored the symptoms and kept going. Then it got worse." She looked up at me. We had just completed the Hundred, a signature Pilates warm-up abdominal exercise that gets your blood circulating from head to toe. Roseanne's cheeks were flushed. "There was no question of working then," she continued. "It took all morning to get out of bed. And when I did—seriously—I could not walk across the room. It was like someone had pulled out my plug."

Before Roseanne had ground herself into an exhausted, bedridden state, she had devoted ten years to indulging her two passions: work and being a perfectionist. Roseanne described a career in sales that at first went very well for her. It meant long hours during the day and often bringing work home in the evenings. Many of her weekends were used to squeeze in business travel. "It was a heady time," she told me. She worked for a small company; everyone had a cut in the business and they were all making a great deal of money. She lost one significant relationship over her need to install a fax at a vacation home and let that man go without a single backward glance.

Before Roseanne got sick she spent every spare moment in the gym exhausting her body with heavy weights. Building her body was the one thing over which she felt control. It was also a way to have power over how she was perceived by others. "So much in my life was about winning," she told me. "And being perfect."

I nodded silently. How many ventures had I taken on with the voice of perfectionism breathing down my neck? The pursuit of perfectionism is a vice deeply embedded in many of us. This self-destructive, obsessive mind-space hounds the afflicted every waking moment. Roseanne was smarter than most. After she got sick she not only walked away forever from an extremely lucrative yet unmerciful job but found a talented therapist who got her to focus on both the external *and* the internal stresses that caused her body to break down. The therapist was convinced that understanding both levels was essential to Roseanne's recovery. Now in the certification program, whenever she got praised for her teaching skills or for her exquisite body, Roseanne would pull herself back from identifying too closely with the compliment. For Roseanne, balancing stress became a process of looking at the emotional baggage she carried around inside—not focusing on just the more obvious outer stresses.

Roseanne told me that the first thing she did when she returned home after being certified was to remove all the mirrors from her Pilates studio. I found this an amazing act. Roseanne e-mailed me: "I want to be guided from the inside, not the outside."

Stress

Stress is the body's survival mechanism against what it perceives as danger. This "danger" can be anything that puts pressure on an individual physically or emotionally. The most obvious stresses come from the outside: change of job or marital status, illness, and financial problems. The more covert stresses linger deeply buried.

Anger and anxiety is generated by stress, and because we all have a tendency to repress unpleasant or painful emotions, these strong emotions build up. They may live for a very long time buried in the subconscious. Roseanne thought she was coping well with the stress of her sales job. She told me this more than once: how proud she and her family were that she rose to the occasion and became the most hardworking and hyperresponsible member of her family. She was extremely good at keeping up a facade at business meetings and hiding anger and frustration at the amount of work doled out to her.

Mainstream researchers have begun to document what people have always suspected: stressful lives actually trigger a biochemical chain of events that affects the body. Because chronic stress can compromise the body's immune system and lead to serious disease, more and more health plans are covering visits to massage and relaxation clinics.

In chapter 2 we discussed how "breathers," or relaxation poses, are built into the Pilates on the Ball workout, as they should be in our ordinary lives. Yet there are other methods that manage stress, burnout, and our perpetually changing inner weather and moods.

A Visit to a Relaxation Clinic and Other Stress Releasers

I remember my first visit to a relaxation clinic. I had just moved to Toronto, a large city where I knew no one, after living for almost thirteen years outside of Canada. I brought to that clinic a certain cynicism—a deep chip on my shoulder—that I thought could never be dissolved or released. I had spent the last few years in Africa, and though I had not even begun to integrate that experience, my world had been utterly changed by it. Here I was lying fully clothed under blankets on table-beds alongside fifteen others while New Age music tinkled above us. We were told to visualize the sun and the surf, and I thought of poverty and apartheid. We were told to imagine our bodies dissolving into sand, and my body ached for people who had touched me deeply, whom I may never see again. I felt utterly alone on that table-bed and, in spite of the blankets, utterly cold. Was it a mistake to return to Canada? Was it a mistake ever to have left?

123

depression and exercise

Regular exercise is an effective antidote to many of the ravages of stress, but lately it has been linked to controlling depression.

Last year Duke University recruited a group of men and women who suffered from serious depression and found out that for some people exercise worked as well as drugs. "Exercise is a viable alternative to drugs," said lead researcher James Blumenthal. "It may not be for everyone, but if a patient is motivated, the chance of beating depression (through exercise) may actually be better."

Over the weeks, Dorothy Madgett, a blind therapist with a gentle voice, urged us to focus on our breath as it moved in and out of the body. Then she took us through a guided visualization where we released one body part at a time. The touch of her hands on the back of my neck lasted only for a few seconds, but to this day I remember how sweetly it penetrated my body. I also recall the startling release of her "laugh therapy." My irritation with New Age jargon and complete strangers disappeared. I went to that clinic weekly for four months and was eventually able to replace images of anxiety and depression with peace and quiet. I got a glimpse that coming home had been the right decision.

Our reactions are linked to our thoughts. Visualizing a beautiful beach or other pleasant scene releases the body. Snapshot moments return to us and remind us how wonderful our lives are. Distance is achieved and we forget and forgive. Relaxation clinics also teach bed exercises—simple movements to be performed in your bed when insomnia strikes and you find your mind spinning off in a million directions.

Massage is excellent preventive medicine that I have enjoyed many times in my life. Massage is known to be very effective for releasing the body of physical and emotional tension. It is also great for improving circulation and stimulating the lymphatic drainage system. Shiatsu, which is based on Chinese acupuncture meridians, is a form of Japanese massage where the pads of the thumbs are applied to various pressure points over the entire body. It is very deep work and can take a few sessions for newcomers to be receptive to its power. Reflexology is a treatment that involves pressure-point touch for hands and feet. Parts of the foot or the hand correspond to internal organs elsewhere in the body. The reflexologist, like the Shiatsu therapist, stimulates these organs to promote healing and clear energy blockages.

Meditation is a journey that your mind takes toward serenity. Meditation can be a difficult journey for most because we often find it torturous to just sit and be. A course in meditation will instruct you how to explore its complexities and experience its benefits. Meditation teaches you to empty your mind of not only deadlines and shopping lists, but also judgments, conflicts, stress, and fears, and to simply experience the present moment.

Breath is key in all these therapies. It is also crucial in most mind/body exercise methods. Slow, smooth breathing calms us and focuses the mind. We hold tension in our bodies in different ways; deep breathing can make us aware of where we are holding stress. It also focuses the mind inward. One of the most dramatic aspects of mind/body exercise is how you can arrive at a class in a total state of agitation and afterward not have a care in the world.

The Cardiovascular Exercises

Cardiovascular exercise reduces stress and increases the oxygen flow to the brain and heart. It also decreases blood pressure and cholesterol and helps you lose weight. Some believe that if you work with intensity a Pilates workout can be a cardiovascular workout, but this function is usually out of the scope of the Pilates Method. However, enhancing or restoring cardiovascular function is an important component of fitness. Although the following exercises are not part of the Pilates Method, I believe strongly that they belong in a book devoted to the exercise ball and overall wellness.

I attribute much of my general knowledge of the exercise ball to physical therapist Joanne Posner-Mayer. Her books and videos have inspired me when selecting the following bouncing-on-the-ball exercises. I have also consulted the videos of Fitball masters Trish Scott and Cheryl Soleway for ideas of cardiovascular exercises (see the resources section).

These exercises will not only increase your heart rate but also help you to work out safely. The ball cushions the body and will automatically activate the appropriate muscles to support the spine. Joanne Posner-Mayer asserts that bouncing on the ball helps to align the spine and activates the muscles around the spine to tighten and support it, and that bouncing for extended periods can increase postural endurance for unsupported sitting and standing. Enjoy yourself as you release stress and enhance cardiovascular fitness at the same time.

Follow these guidelines when bouncing on the ball.

- Work in good posture.

- Never bend or twist the spine when bouncing.

- Be sure that you have enough space or use a nearby chair to help with balance. Newcomers to the ball should keep one hand on the ball when starting.

- At the height of your cardiovascular workout, always maintain enough wind to be able to carry on a conversation.

- Do not forget to build a cooldown section into your aerobic workout. Do not simply stop. Instead, continue to bounce gently with slow and easy arm movements, not above heart level.

- To protect knees and hips, aerobic teachers prefer a larger ball for a lot of bouncing work. The angle at the hip should not exceed 90 degrees.

aerobic exercise

Aerobic exercise should be part of any exercise program, but you should avoid high-impact exercises. Working on the ball is an optimal medium because it cushions the body. Problems can increase if correct posture is not maintained. Start a cardiovascular program at a moderate intensity of fifteen minutes three times a week.

125

Bouncing Plus

Bounce as vigorously as you can, but take care that you don't bounce off the ball. You may want to start by touching a piece of furniture to keep balance. These exercises can be intensified by using small weights or bouncing in double-time. Repeated bouncing, with or without arm and leg movements, will increase the heart rate, but only if these activities are sustained long enough.

Purpose To warm up the body and improve cardiovascular fitness and coordination.

Watchpoints • Do not bend or twist the spine while bouncing. • Keep the neck and head aligned on the spine. • Keep toes and knees aligned. Do not let knees project beyond the toes.

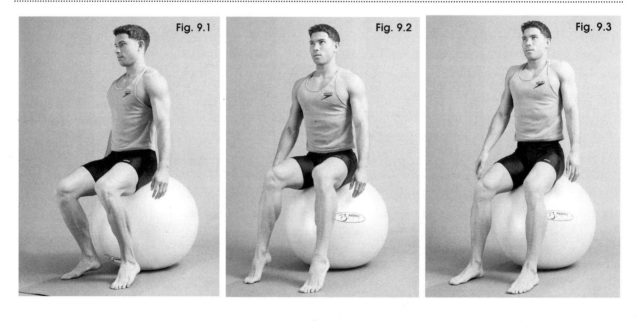

Fig. 9.1   Fig. 9.2   Fig. 9.3

starting position

Sit on the center of your ball, knees aligned with ankles, legs just wider than hip-distance apart, feet parallel.

movement 1: bouncing

Press feet to the floor, activate the thigh muscles, and bounce as vigorously as is comfortable (fig. 9.1). Relax and breathe as you bounce.

movement 2: heel raises

Press the toes into the floor and lift the heels as you bounce (fig. 9.2).

movement 3: shoulder shrugs

1. As you bounce, lift and lower the shoulders (fig. 9.3).
2. Repeat each move eight to ten times, and gradually build up the repetitions.

Bouncing with Arms

Practice these following exercises first without bouncing. Holding one-pound weights in your hands can enhance all of these exercises, but take care to keep your feet planted on the floor for the first three exercises. Balance and coordination are challenged and the cardiovascular system is taxed when arm swings are added to the bounce.

Purpose To warm up the body and improve cardiovascular fitness and coordination.

Watchpoints • Practice first with the feet on the ground. • Keep arms within a comfortable range. • Keep knees in line with feet. • Keep arms low if you have neck problems.

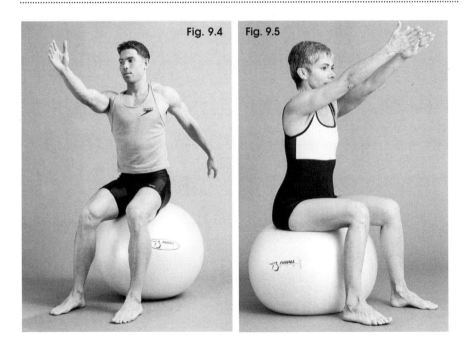

Fig. 9.4   Fig. 9.5

starting position

Sit on the center of your ball, knees over ankles, legs just wider than hip-distance apart, feet parallel.

movement 1: arm swings

Move one arm forward, the other backward (fig. 9.4). Swing the arms.

Then press feet to the floor, activate the thigh muscles, and bounce. Move one arm forward, the other back.

movement 2: clap front and back

As you bounce, clap your hands in front of your body (fig. 9.5) and then behind.

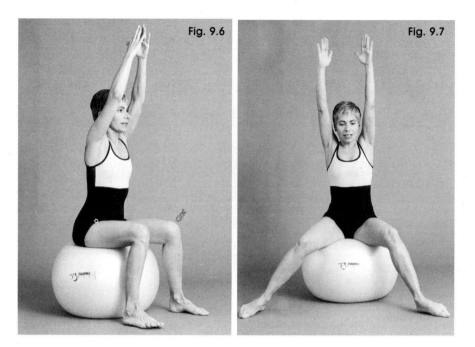

Fig. 9.6

Fig. 9.7

movement 3: clap overhead

As you bounce, clap your hands overhead (fig. 9.6) and then on the side of the ball.

movement 4: jumping janes— intermediate

1. Try arms only first. As you bounce clap your hands overhead. With the next bounce return to center and clap hands on the side of the ball.

2. Add legs: as you bounce open your legs and clap your hands overhead (fig. 9.7).

3. With the next bounce clap hands on the side of the ball and return legs to center.

4. Repeat each move eight to ten times.

Foot Taps

You may want to try this first without bouncing. Lifting the foot reduces the base of support and makes you work hard to stay on the ball. When you have mastered the front and side taps, try can-can steps, parallel skiing moves, or any bouncing combination your heart desires. Arm movements can be added, but when you lift the arms to the side keep them below shoulder height. This helps to keep the shoulders down. Don't forget to monitor your heart rate.

Purpose To warm up the body and improve cardiovascular fitness and coordination.

Watchpoint • Relax and breathe as you bounce.

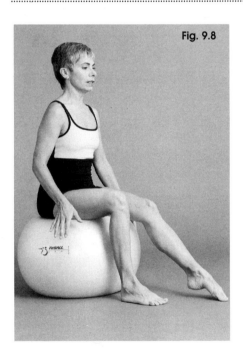

Fig. 9.8

starting position

1. Sit on the center of your ball, knees over ankles, legs just wider than hip-distance apart, feet parallel.
2. Press the feet to the floor, activate the thigh muscles, and bounce.

movement 1: front foot tap

1. On the first bounce, tap one foot in front of you (fig. 9.8). With the next bounce, return foot to start.
2. Repeat eight to ten times on each side and gradually build up the repetitions.

movement 2: side foot tap

1. On the first bounce, tap one foot to the side. With the next bounce, return foot to center.
2. Repeat eight to ten times on each side and gradually build up the repetitions.

Foot Kicks

Cleverness is in the air with these kicks. Maintain good posture as you lift the leg; eye gaze is straight ahead. Adding arms to leg movements challenges coordination, timing, and balance.

Purpose To warm up the body and improve cardiovascular fitness and coordination.

Watchpoint • Be sure that good postural alignment is not compromised by your movement.

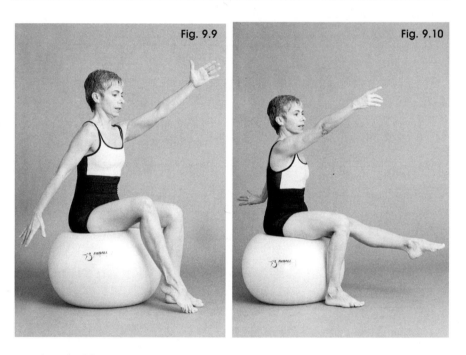

Fig. 9.9   Fig. 9.10

starting position

1. Sit on the center of your ball, knees over ankles, legs just wider than hip-distance apart, feet parallel.
2. Press feet to the floor, activate the thigh muscles, and bounce.

movement 1: marches

1. With one bounce, lift up one knee. With the next bounce place the foot down.
2. Repeat with the other foot and continue marching.

3. Add arms, opposite arm to leg (fig. 9.9).

movement 2: kicks

1. With one bounce kick one foot up until the knee is as straight as possible. With the next bounce, return the foot to the floor.
2. Repeat with the other leg and continue kicking.
3. Add arms, opposite arm to leg (fig. 9.10).
4. Repeat each move eight to ten times and gradually build up the repetitions.

Moving around the Ball

The following exercises are much harder than they look. Take care not to roll into furniture or other objects in the room. Cushion your landing with the feet. Remember: you are moving the body on the upward part of the bounce.

Purpose To warm up the body and improve cardiovascular fitness and coordination.

Watchpoint • Be sure that good postural alignment is not compromised by your movement.

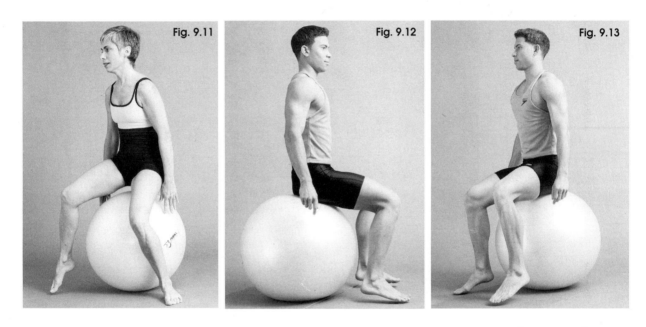

Fig. 9.11   Fig. 9.12   Fig. 9.13

starting position

1. Sit on the center of your ball, knees over ankles, legs just wider than hip-distance apart, feet parallel.
2. Press feet to the floor, activate the thigh muscles, and bounce.

movement 1: step around—intermediate

1. Bounce and step one foot sideways (fig. 9.11). With the next bounce, bring the other foot to meet it.
2. Repeat as you circle the ball.
3. Reverse the direction.

movement 2: hop around—intermediate

1. Bounce and hop both feet to the side (fig. 9.12).
2. Repeat hopping as you circle the ball in one direction (fig. 9.13).
3. Reverse the direction.
4. Repeat two or three times in each direction.

De-stressing on the Ball

Many of the exercises found in a modern aerobics class can be transported safely to the ball. No more excuses for boredom or forcefully pushing yourself to keep pedaling that extra mile on a stationary bike. But there are many other ways of releasing stress. In any workout, a balance between exertion and total relaxation needs to be struck.

Now we slow things down and use the ball not to bounce on but to foster release and repose. Sometimes the first step in letting go of stress is simply being able to recognize when we are holding tension. The next step is learning to experience a deep state of relaxation so that we can return to it when necessary. Resting after a workout is highly beneficial, but do not use the relaxation poses as your cooldown after an intense aerobic workout such as running or bicycle racing. These poses should occur only after cooling down. Or enjoy them on their own as breathers or relaxation intervals after a stressful day.

In relaxation pose 1, slipping the ball under your knees releases the lower back from undue stress. A small flat pillow under the head may make you more comfortable. If your feet are cold, wear socks. Have a blanket nearby.

Some people do not find it relaxing to lie on their backs. If that is true for you, then you might want to try relaxation pose 2. Most people love this pose: not only does it open the upper spine and release the neck muscles but it gives one the sensation of womblike safety and comfort. If you get motion sickness, kneel before the ball, kick one knee in and then the other, and hug the ball, releasing the head to one side.

In relaxation pose 3 half the body is turned upside down, creating a powerful energizing effect. Adapted from a yoga posture, this pose can help cleanse the organs and heal a fierce headache. It's also a great remedy for sore legs and achy feet. Whenever fatigue strikes, put your feet up for a while and refresh yourself.

Sometimes just lying on the floor doing nothing is the most challenging "exercise" of all, because our minds are always overworking and are easily distracted. De-stressing on the ball is open to anyone, no matter what your fitness level. If you can breathe you can relax. Remember: we are trying to release the mind as well as the body.

relaxation pose 1

1. Slip the ball under your knees and settle your lower back into the floor (fig. 9.14). Allow your eyelids to close and then let the eyeballs sink effortlessly into their sockets. Focus on your breath, especially on the long exhale, and the overall feeling of ease that it brings to the body.

2. Now make a tight fist with your right hand, hold for four counts, and release.

3. Stretch your right hand back at the wrist, hold for four counts, and release.

4. Raise your right hand up to your shoulder, squeeze for four counts, and release.

5. Stretch your right toes back into flexion, hold for four counts, and release.

6. Tighten your right calf muscles by pushing them into the ball, hold for four counts, and release.

7. Lift your right leg off the ball two inches, hold for four counts, and drop it on the ball.

8. Lift your right buttock one inch off the mat, squeeze for four counts, and release.

9. Bring your right shoulder up to your ears, hold for four counts, and release.

10. Repeat on the other side of the body.

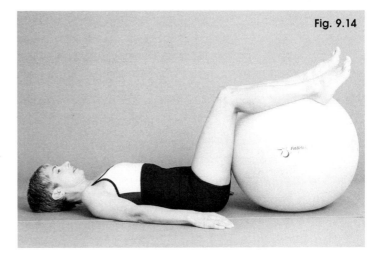

Fig. 9.14

relaxation pose 2

1. Kneel before your ball and drape your body over it, hands on the mat in front of you (fig. 9.15). Allow gravity to naturally stretch your neck and spine as you explore the ball's roundness and air-filled texture.

2. Go deeper so that your head is one inch from the ground.

3. Starting with the little toe of your left foot, bring your awareness to that toe, and then work from toe to toe, heel to arch, arch to ankle, moving along the left foot. Continue to bring your awareness to your left heel, ankle, calf, back of knee, thigh, pelvis, and work up the left side of the body to the torso, arms, and head.

4. Work one side of the body and then the other.

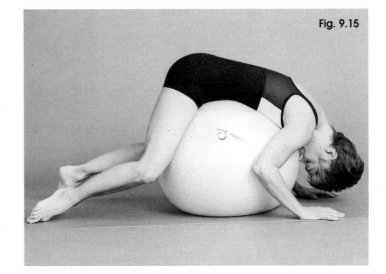

Fig. 9.15

133

relaxation pose 3

1. Scoot your buttocks so you are resting close to a wall. Place the ball against the wall, then slowly roll the ball up the wall with your feet. Balance the ball as much as you can on the soles, not the sides, of your feet. Feet are sitzbone distance apart (fig. 9.16). Hold this position for a few moments, taking some deep easy breaths. Notice how the gentle weight of the ball allows the legs to sink heavy into the hip sockets.

2. Next, push all the breath out, searching for the bottom of the exhale. Find it, explore it, and do not rush into the inhale. Exhale again slowly in this manner.

3. Then practice breathing into the back of the rib cage. Feel the back of the ribs open and close on the mat.

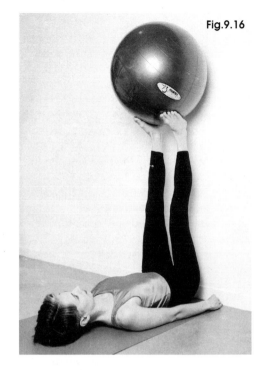

Fig.9.16

4. Finally, try breathing deep into the belly, noticing how the pelvis muscles release.

5. As the blood rushes down the legs, feel the release.

6. Hold this position for 5 minutes or so, using breath to coax tension out of the body.

In the next chapter I have detailed three different workouts: Basic Ball, Intermediate Ball and, for those of you recovering from injuries or limitations, Restorative Ball. I've designed these workouts to meet different fitness needs and expectations.

I predict that during this decade the world is going to have a big love affair with the exercise ball. Join us and be a part of that love affair.

10

Pilates on the Ball for Life

Journeys versus Arrivals: Lucy's Story

Five years ago Lucy was diagnosed with multiple sclerosis. Even though it is not immediately life threatening, multiple sclerosis can be vicious in the way it selects and destroys areas of the brain and spinal cord and leaves the sufferer fearful as to how the disease may play itself out in the body. Symptoms include weakness; sensory deficits; and balance, vision, and bladder problems.

I was not sure how much I could help Lucy. As with so many injuries and diseases, you need to balance research about the condition with your experience of what you actually see when working with a person. I agreed to give it a try.

Joseph Pilates's method of physical and mental conditioning was originally called Contrology. Pilates wanted students to gain mastery over their minds and their bodies. For all of us, especially Lucy, that means working within our limitations.

Lucy's goal was to keep as much mobility as possible so that she could be independent and not have to rely too much on her wheelchair. She also wanted to get muscle tone back in her legs and to improve her stability when moving as much as possible. The weakness in her legs was greater on one side, and she spoke about feeling nauseous when she could not connect the sensation of the bottoms of her feet to her body.

When we began to work together I noticed that Lucy wanted to hurry and finish each set of reps. I felt her "jerkiness" was not simply the result of decreased muscle tone or the difficulty of coordinating the sequence of movements. It was almost as if her mind were telling her body to race to the rapid beat of some aerobics class of the past. She also insisted on knowing how many reps and how many sets of each exercise we should do. She was surprised when I explained that we would only do one set of six to eight reps. She had been forcing herself to do three sets of ten reps no matter how much she hated the exercise. This kind of strict force-feeding—whether it is to look good in a tank top or, in Lucy's case, to save her body from loss of function—can translate into a deep hatred of gyms, exercise equipment, and exercise in general.

Like many people Lucy was astonished to hear that effective results could be achieved by not overworking the body. I also reminded her that overworking was counterproductive for someone with MS, where fatigue levels must be constantly monitored throughout the day.

In the next session I gently broached the subject of Lucy's attitude toward exercise. Lucy confessed what I already suspected: that she disliked exercise and had done so all her life. She was not interested in learning about the Pilates Method or exploring ballwork for its own sake but only as a means of getting to her destination—an improvement in her muscle tone.

I could not imagine what the day-to-day management of this unpredictable disease would be like. But I did sympathize with Lucy's attitude. Like many people I am very goal-oriented and want quick solutions and fixes to my problems, big or small. I am also in a tremendous hurry to arrive, even though experience has shown me again and again that true satisfaction lies in the journey: the acceptance of life at the present moment. As many a weary traveler has discovered, arriving is not all that it is cut out to be.

Fortunately, Lucy liked the idea of the ball. She saw it as playful and fun. We were both hoping that the ball would inspire her through the valleys and hills that were ahead.

We started with breath. The breathing did not come easily and we spent a great deal of time on it. "It's all right," I assured Lucy as she flicked her eyes to the clock. "The breath is part of what we need to learn." I explained that the breath helps the body let go and surrender to the immediate moment. I believe this is one of the key reasons it takes people so long to feel comfortable with breathwork. We breathe every second of the day but we do not easily open ourselves to living and accepting the here and now.

In the third session I suggested we change rooms. At the time her exercise room was a fluorescently lit room shared by a freezer, an old walker, and a graveyard of various pieces of equipment that Lucy confessed she never used. The walls were lined with exercise tapes that she had purchased but had never even taken out of their plastic wrappers. I suggested we move in to another room, one that she could associate with relaxation and pleasure and not with failed exercise attempts from the past.

Over the weeks Lucy discovered that there was something to be found in each of the exercises themselves. Sometimes that meant simply feeling the movement on her good side and then comparing that to her weak side. Some days the signals were not getting through to her body, but her muscles still had the capacity to work, so we did passive stretching or breathwork. I kept her focused on what we were accomplishing day to day. It was a hard-won goal, but eventually Lucy saw the value of exercise for itself, not just as something she had to do. I admired Lucy for the courage it took for her to accept this decision.

Honor Your Own Pace

No one can define how rapid your fitness improvement should be. There are many fitness books and magazine articles offering clues to other peoples' athletic marathons and warrior weekends, but each case is different. A mind/body journey is as private as any solo voyage. Agents of change—coaches, trainers, well-wishers, and fellow travelers—can only give you so much advice. The journey is a solitary one: when you reach plateaus or dips it is only you who can maneuver through them. It is only you who wins the rewards.

What I love about the ball is that it is unpredictable and playful and encourages you to dig deeply within yourself to cope with it. Remember: growth comes to us in fits and starts. There may be a long plateau of frustration when progress doesn't appear to happen. We all have those days when we want to give up—to let the air out of the ball and store it away. Please don't do this! On those days give yourself permission to be lazy. Do a few stretches over the ball and then ease into a delicious relaxation pose. You may want to accompany this by deep breathing or playing a guided imagery tape. Or shift gears and simply sit on the ball while you watch television or speak on the phone. Ten minutes of ball sitting is good for the back and talking to a friend will clear the air.

Luckily one of the best aspects of Pilates on the Ball is that most students feel taller and stronger even after one session. Suddenly you will enjoy performing an exercise, such as push ups, for example, which you never thought you would do again in your life. You will notice that your waistband feels looser, your thighs leaner, and that your arms and back are strong and sculpted.

Accept Yourself as You Are Today

In the introduction we discussed the importance of healing your relationship with physical activity. I hope this book has led you closer to understanding your body and your psychological connection to exercise. By gaining this understanding you can move ahead and reap the benefits of Pilates on the Ball whether you are very fit or deconditioned. Part of the solution is a balance between accepting where your body is and then gently, yet firmly, inspiring it to go further.

When I studied ballet I often focused on what I was not. A voice in my head could not be silenced: I began too late, I was not as flexible or as skinny as the other dancers, I mixed up the choreography, my jumps were without grace, my pirouettes too unwieldy. I loved the physical sensation of dancing—the sensual rush of flying through space—but I poisoned those longings with constantly comparing myself to others. This hostility caused a bottomless pit of longings, envies, and neediness. When I got the wonderful opportunity to study with a prestigious teacher or attend a special ballet school in the summer, anxiety and shame destroyed the pleasure of these experiences. Dance, which had started off as a friend, ended up as an enemy that had this power to make me happy or sad, self-loving or self-hating.

Stop right now and take an inventory of all the physical joys that your life now possesses. List them in your mind or on a piece of paper: your health, your mobility, the power of being able to walk, to see the beauty around you. If you have a long-term chronic condition or some other serious disease that has affected your nervous system, try to focus on what mobility you possess and what realistic goals can be set to nurture your strength, endurance, and coordination. Don't forget your physical accomplishments of the past. Your body will remember where you were before and may get you back there quicker than you might imagine possible. Ponder your personal well-being— how good it feels to be in *your* skin and not anybody else's. Don't resent your body for its years of being sedentary, or fight its tightness or restrictions. Don't despise its weaknesses, its pains, bulges, and diseases. Accept yourself as you are today.

Three Workouts

I leave you with three workouts: Restorative Ball, a gentle workout for those recovering from injuries or returning to exercise; Basic Ball, for those of you who are just beginning but have no limitations or injuries; and Intermediate

Perform your work with minimum effort and maximum pleasure.

—Joseph Pilates

Ball, for those of you who are strong and fit and have successfully mastered Basic Ball. If you are just beginning, start with Restorative Ball and work up to Basic Ball and eventually Intermediate Ball.

Each workout is a complete session in itself. Try to complete the whole workout if you can, or at least sections of it—each level is set up like a complete dance from which you cannot just abstract a few steps. Stretching throughout the workout and at the end will gently break down scar tissue. Remember the principles of Pilates when you perform this work. You are engaging the mind and controlling the body with precise yet effortless movement. Practice will help you master the moves. Pay attention to the watchpoints and your body's messages. Notice the exercises that you instinctively turn away from. Sometimes we resist the exercises that we need the most. Once you have mastered the basic skills you can add the elements of flow and intensity to your workout.

Remember it is not only the exercises that are important but the philosophies and principles behind the method. The ability to center your life and balance daily stresses will maintain good health in your mind and body. Precision, alertness, and focus, not to forget proper breathing and posture, should extend into all parts of your life. If you keep in touch with the meaning behind the gesture, whether it is cross-stitching a quilt or draping your body over a ball, the benefits and rewards will multiply.

The time to embrace Pilates on the Ball for life is now. So often we participate in healing our mind and bodies only after something goes wrong. Get out of the rut of overworking and build in time for relaxation and fun. Make changes now to revive your humor and your immune syusystem. Take an honest look at how good you are to yourself and recall Chi Ball practitioner Monica Linford's timely words: "Would you starve, neglect, or overwork your best friend? Then why do it to yourself?"

Each workout here has been laid out with thumbnail photos to provide a quick reference. One photo has been shown to represent each movement and to visibly trigger your memory of the exercise. The page numbers are supplied so you can easily cross-reference back to the full instructions in the text. The top name is the exercise name with its corresponding page number; under it is the movement name and the order in which the exercises should be followed. Remember, you are free to do sections of the workout, if desired, but try and follow the exercises in order as much as possible.

Start with three sessions a week—even if all you do is twenty to thirty

basic principles: a review

The following principles of the Pilates Method are the bedrock on which Pilates on the Ball is built.

Concentration—engage your mind on what your body is doing.

Control—foster mind/body coordination that guarantees that movements will not be sloppy or haphazard.

Centering—work from a strong core.

Breathing—breathe into the rib cage.

Postural alignment—be aware of the position of your body parts in space.

Flow—move slowly and gracefully.

Precision—move with exact, efficient, accurate body strokes.

Stamina—when you are ready, introduce the element of intensity to build endurance.

Relaxation—learn to release the body and not overwork it.

minutes each time. Schedule regular workouts into your routine, even write them into your day planner, to keep you on track and make your ballwork a priority. Are you a morning person? Or will you have the discipline at night to workout at your gym or at home alone? It is strongly advised that you consult your health care practitioner before starting this or any new exercise program.

WORKOUT 1:
Restorative Ball

Restorative Ball

The goal of this workout is to move the body and strengthen it without aggravating or reinjuring it. Restorative Ball is a gentle workout that can alleviate some of the pain of arthritis and lower back injury. It can relax stiff muscles and joints, but only if you work cautiously and slowly. Be aware of your limitations. Remember: we are not simply trying to fix the problem area. We are trying to strengthen the muscles and joints around the area, and we are also trying to work in good posture and alignment. We want to strengthen the abdominals and other core muscles and add flexibility to the body.

If you have a sore neck keep your head on the mat when possible and do the abdominal exercises without the ball, placing your hands behind your neck to support it whenever you lift the head off the mat. It is essential to check with your health care practitioner about these exercises before you begin; you may want to take this book in to show her or him.

Sitting (p. 32)

1. sitting

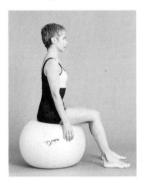

2. pelvic tilt

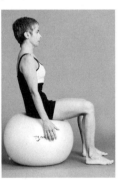

Bouncing (p. 34)

3. gentle bouncing

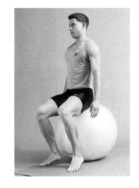

Bouncing Plus (p. 126)

4. heel raises

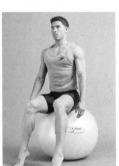

5. shoulder shrugs

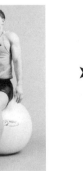

Foot Taps (p. 129)

6. front foot tap/side foot tap

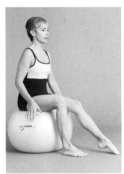

Foot Kicks (p. 130)

7. marches

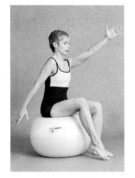

(legs only at first,
then add arms)

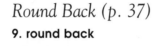

Stop Bouncing

➤

Spine Stretch Forward (p. 35)

8. spine stretch forward

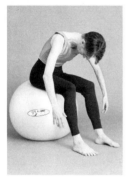

Round Back (p. 37)

9. round back

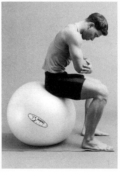

Spine Twist (p. 39)

10. spine twist

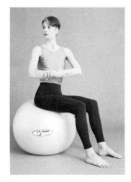

(keep this rotation small;
think of lengthening
the spine, not rotating)

Go to the Mat

➤

Breathing Observations (p. 22)

11. abdominal breathing

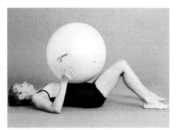

12. rib cage breathing

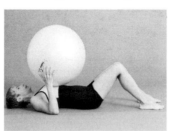

Little Abdominal Curls (p. 48)

13. little abdominal curls

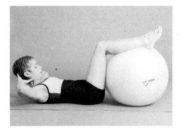

Full Abdominal Curls (p. 49)

14. full abdominal curls

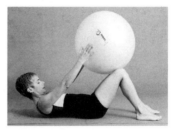

The Rollup (p. 52)

15. half rollup

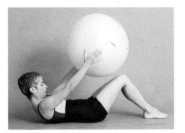

(keep knees bent)

Leg Circles (p. 54)

16. leg circles

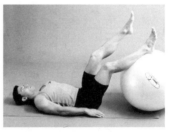

Single Leg Stretch (p. 56)

17. single leg stretch

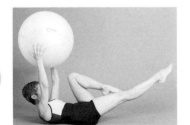

(leave head on mat and keep
legs very high in the air)

Obliques (p. 58)

18. just squeeze

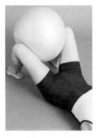

Hip Rolls (p. 93)
19. hip rolls

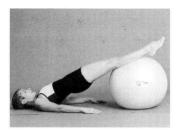

(keep very small)

Hip Lift (p. 97)
20. hip lift

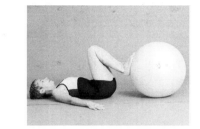

(keep pelvis on the mat as you roll the ball in and out)

On the Side (p. 100)
21. on the side

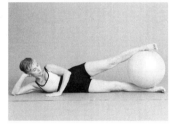

(just squeeze ball between legs, do not lift legs)

Belly on the Ball

Navel-to-Spine (p. 46)
22. navel-to-spine

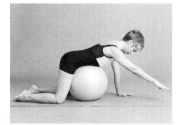

The Swan (p. 63)
23. the swan

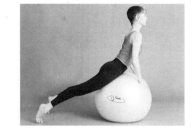

(keep this extension very small)

The Push-up (p. 102)

24. basic push-up

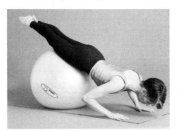

(keep movement small and lift
abdominals to protect lower back)

De-stressing on the Ball (p. 132)

25. relaxation pose two

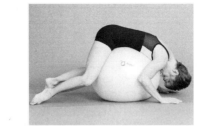

➤

Sit on the Ball ➤

Hug a Tree (p. 75)

26. hug a tree

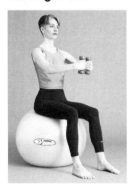

(avoid if you have
round shoulders)

Open Shoulders and Biceps Curl (p. 76)

27. open shoulders   **28. biceps curl**

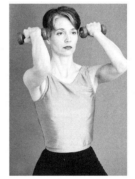 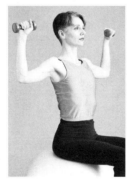

➤

Salute (p. 77)

29. salute

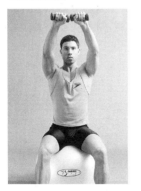

➤

Rowing (p. 78)

30. rowing

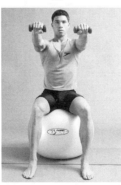

➤

Stand at the Wall ➤

Footwork Exercises (p. 81)

31. parallel feet **32. small turnout** **33. high half toe** **34. wide squat**

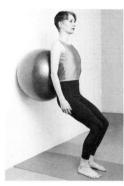 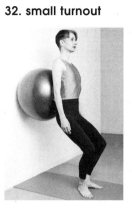 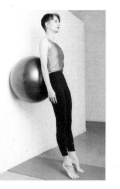 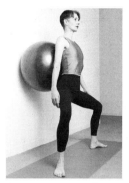

➤

➤ **Stretches** ➤

Shoulder Stretches (p. 117)

35. shoulder shrug **36. arms overhead** **37. interlaced fingers**

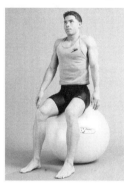 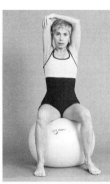 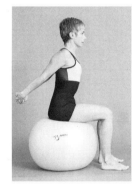

➤

Frog Stretch (p. 110)
38. frog stretch

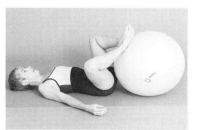

➤

Hamstring Stretch (p. 111)
39. hamstring stretch with towel

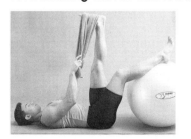

➤

147

Hip Stretch (p. 112)
40. hip stretch

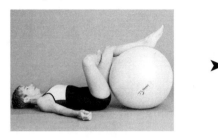

Neck Stretch (p. 113)
41. neck stretch

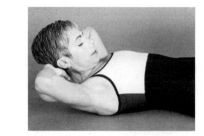

De-stressing on the Ball (p. 132)
42. relaxation pose 1

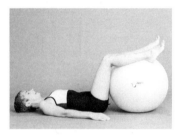

WORKOUT 2:
Basic Ball

Basic Ball

Basic Ball is for those of you who have successfully completed Restorative Ball and have no limitations or injuries. At this level we are trying to gain skills and master the essential work with precision and ease. We want to make sure we are initiating each move with breath and using the breath to move the body as efficiently as possible. We want to continue to strengthen the abdominals and other core muscles and add flexibility to the body. If you have a healthy spine we are going to add full extension, flexion, rotation, and sidebending to your workout.

Sitting (p. 33)

1. sitting

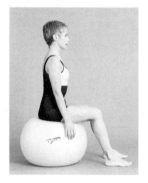

2. pelvic tilt

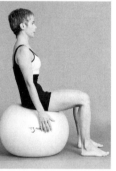

Bouncing (p. 34)

3. gentle bouncing

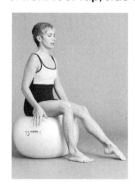

Bouncing Plus (p. 126)

4. heel raises

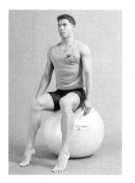

5. shoulder shrugs

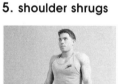

Foot Taps (p. 129)

6. front foot tap/side foot tap

Foot Kicks (p. 130)
7. marches

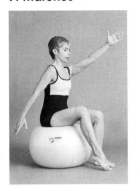

Bouncing with Arms (p. 127)
8. arm swings   **9. clap front and back**   **10. clap overhead**

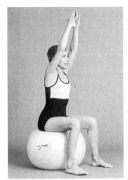

11. jumping janes

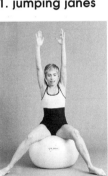

(first without arms)

Stop Bouncing

Spine Stretch Forward (p. 35)
12. spine stretch forward

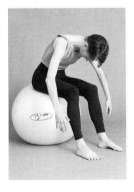

The Saw (p. 36)
13. the saw

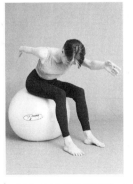

(add hamstring stretch
when ready)

151

Round Back (p. 37)

14. round back

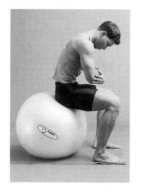

➤

Seated Lateral Shift (p. 38)

15. seated lateral shift

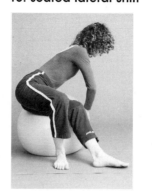

➤

Spine Twist (p. 39)

16. spine twist

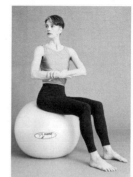

➤

Mermaid (p. 40)

17. mermaid

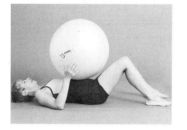

➤

Go to the Mat

➤

Breathing Observations (p. 22)

18. abdominal breathing

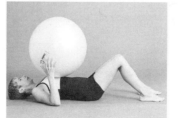

19. rib cage breathing

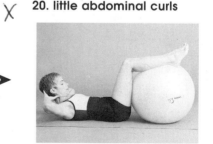

Little Abdominal Curls (p. 48)

20. little abdominal curls

➤

Full Abdominal Curls (p. 49)
21. full abdominal curls

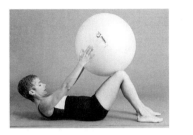

Waterfall (p. 51)
22. waterfall

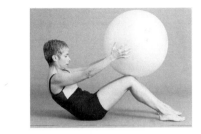

(go as far up as you can)

The Rollup (p. 52)
23. half rollup

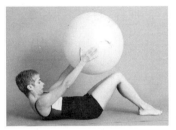

24. full rollup

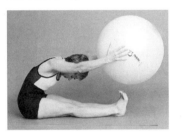

Leg Circles (p. 54)
25. leg circles

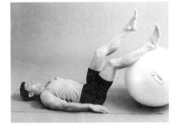

Rolling Like a Ball (p. 55)
26. movement 1

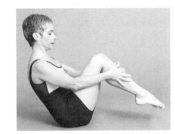

27. movement 2

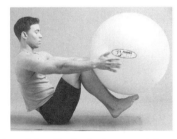

(begin without the ball; advance to adding the ball when ready)

Single Leg Stretch (p. 56)

28. single leg stretch

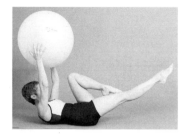

Double Leg Stretch (p. 57)

29. double leg stretch

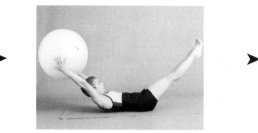

(keep head on the mat if necessary)

Obliques (p. 58)

30. obliques

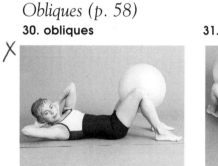

31. just squeeze

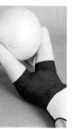

Hip Rolls (p. 92)

32. hip rolls

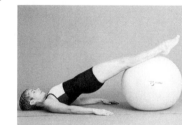

Hip Rolls with Balance (p. 94)

33. hip rolls with balance

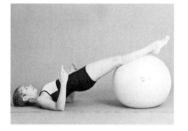

Hip Lift (p. 97)

34. hip lift—intermediate

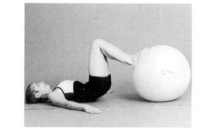

Bend and Stretch (p. 99)

35. bend and stretch

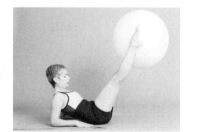

On the Side (p. 100)

36. on the side

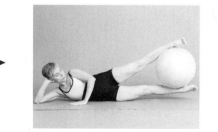

Ball Balance (p. 101)

37. ball balance

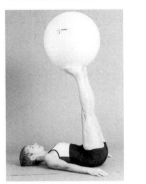

(use the wall if necessary)

➤ | *Belly on the Ball* | ➤

Navel-to-Spine (p. 46)

38. navel-to-spine

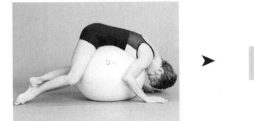

➤

The Swan (p. 63)

39. swan dive

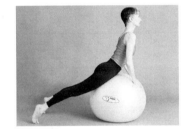

➤

The Push-up (p. 102)

40. push-up

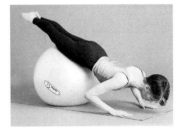

➤

De-stressing on the Ball (p. 132)

41. relaxation pose 2

➤ | *Sit on the Ball* | ➤

Hug a Tree (p. 75)

42. hug a tree

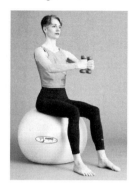

(avoid if you have
round shoulders)

Open Shoulders and Biceps Curls (p. 76)

43. open shoulders

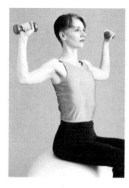

44. biceps curls

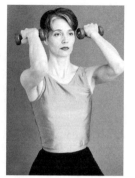

Salute (p. 77)

45. salute

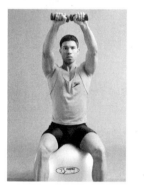

Rowing (p. 78)

46. rowing

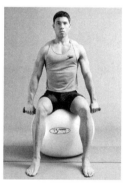

Stand at the Wall

Footwork Exercises (p. 81)

47. parallel feet

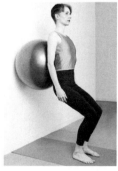

48. small turnout

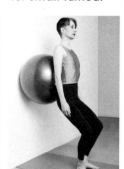

49. high half toe

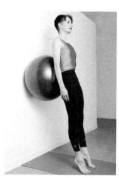

50. lower and lift

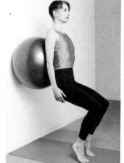

51. wide squat

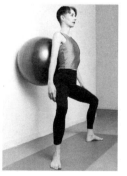

Stretches

Shoulder Stretches (p. 117)

52. shoulder shrug   **53. arms overhead**   **54. interlaced fingers**

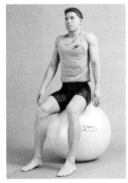 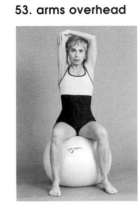 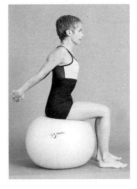

Frog Stretch (p. 110)
55. frog stretch

Hamstring Stretch (p. 111)
56. hamstring stretch with towel

Hip Stretch (p. 112)
57. hip stretch

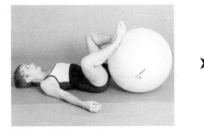 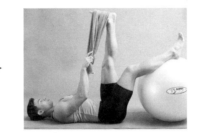 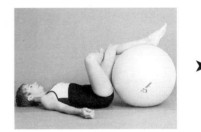

Neck Stretch (p. 113)
58. Neck Stretch

The Shell (p. 114)
59. The Shell

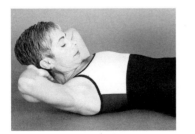 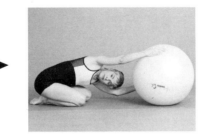

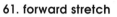

Side Stretches (p. 115)

60. side stretch

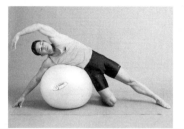

61. forward stretch

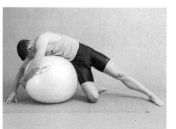

62. chest to ceiling

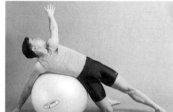

Psoas Stretch (p. 116)

63. psoas stretch

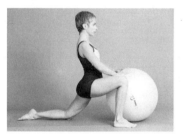

The Arch (p. 118)

64. tabletop

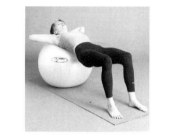

The Squat (p. 120)

65. the squat

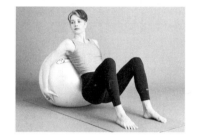

De-stressing on the Ball (p. 132)

66. relaxation pose 2

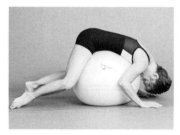

67. relaxation pose 3

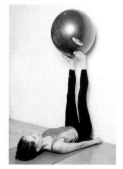

WORKOUT 3:
Intermediate Ball

Intermediate Ball

This workout is for those who are strong, have a sound understanding of Pilates, or a background in dance or athletics, or those who have successfully mastered Basic Ball and want to go further into the work. The goal here is to challenge the body to gain strength without sacrificing technique. Try not to rush the sequence; moving slowly is harder. Occasionally at this level it is appropriate to add the element of speed, but accuracy and precision must remain as stamina is built. Work from a powerful core—remember, it is the small deep muscles that support the larger ones. At an intermediate level we do not necessarily add more weight (though you could work with two-pound weights); we simply challenge our bodies to move precisely and with fluidity. The transitions are as important as the exercises as you move smoothly from one move to the next.

Breathing Observations (p. 22)

1. abdominal breathing   **2. rib cage breathing**

Little Abdominal Curls (p. 48)

3. little abdominal curls

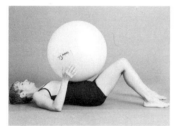
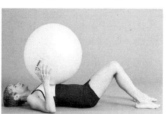
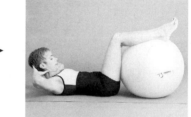

Waterfall (p. 51)

4. waterfall

The Rollup (p. 52)

5. full rollup

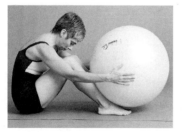
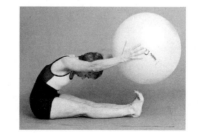

Leg Circles (p. 54)
6. leg circles

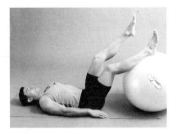

➤

Rolling Like a Ball (p. 55)
7. rolling like a ball

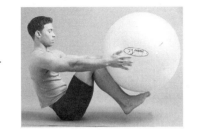

➤

Single Leg Stretch (p. 56)
8. single leg stretch

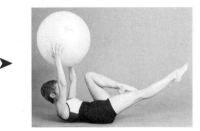

➤

Double Leg Stretch (p. 57)
9. double leg stretch

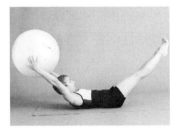

➤

Obliques (p. 58)
10. obliques

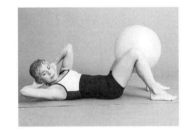

11. just squeeze

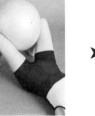

➤

The Rollover (p. 58)
12. the rollover

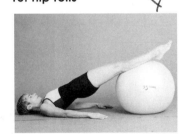

➤

Hip Rolls (p. 93)
13. hip rolls

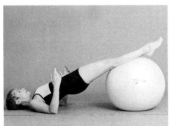

➤

Hip Rolls with Balance (p. 94)
14. basic

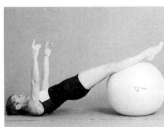

15. intermediate

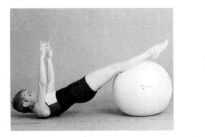

16. advanced

➤

Shoulder Bridges (p. 95)

17. preparation

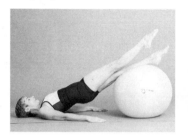

18. full shoulder bridge

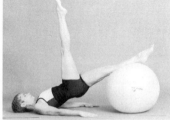

Hip Lift (p. 97)

19. hip lift

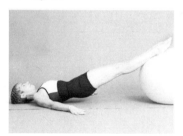

20. one leg hip lift

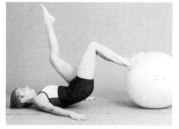

Bend and Stretch (p. 99)

21. bend and stretch

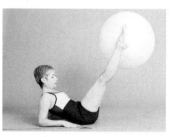

22. ball twist

On the Side (p. 100)

23. on the side

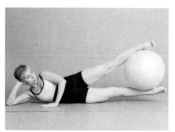

Ball Balance (p. 101)
24. ball balance

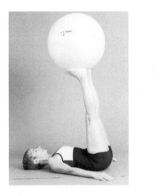

The Push-up (p. 102)
25. the push-up

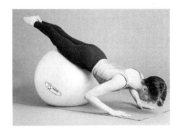

The Pike—Advanced (p. 103)
26. the pike

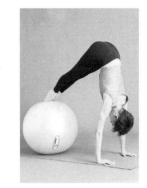

Upper Abdominal Curl (p. 50)
27. upper abdominal curl

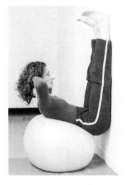

Sit on the Ball

*Spine Stretch
Forward (p. 35)*
28. spine stretch forward

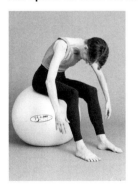

The Saw (p. 36)
29. the saw

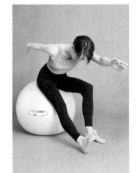

(with hamstring stretch)

Round Back (p. 37)
30. round back

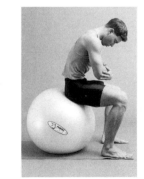

Seated Lateral Shift (p. 38)
31. seated lateral shift

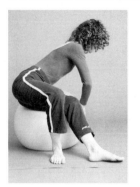

Spine Twist (p. 39)
32. spine twist

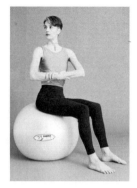

Mermaid (p. 40)
33. mermaid

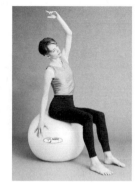

Hug a Tree (p. 75)
34. hug a tree

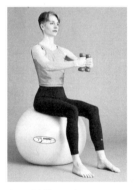

(avoid if you have
round shoulders)

Open Shoulders and Biceps Curls (p. 76)
35. open shoulders   **36. biceps curls**

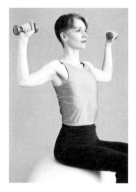 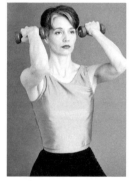

Salute (p. 77)
37. salute

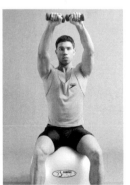

Rowing (p. 78)
38. rowing

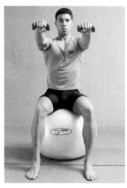

Flies and More Armwork (p. 80)

39. scapula isolation

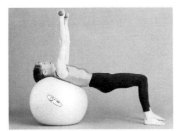

40. chest press

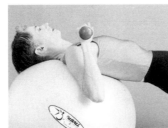

41. flies

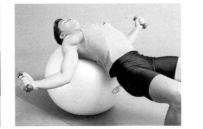

Bouncing Plus (p. 126)

42. heel raises

43. shoulder shrugs

Foot Taps (p. 129)

44. front foot tap/side foot tap

Foot Kicks (p. 130)

45. marches

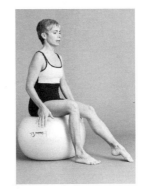

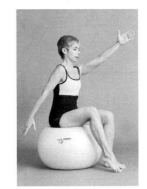

Bouncing with Arms (p. 127)

46. clap overhead

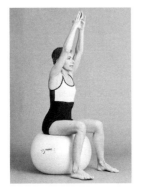

47. clap front and back

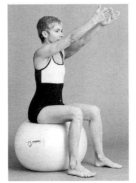

48. jumping janes

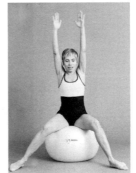

Foot Kicks (p. 130)

49. kicks

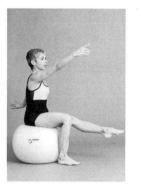

Moving around the Ball (p. 131)

50. step around

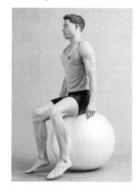

51. hop around

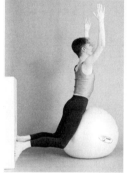

Swan Dive (p. 64)

52. preparation

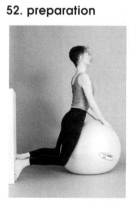

53. full swan dive

Belly on the Ball

Shell on the Ball (p. 66)

54. shell on the ball

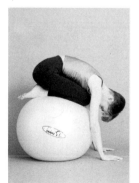

More Extensions (p. 67)

55. open and close legs

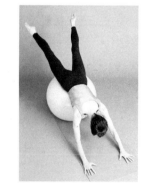

56. beats

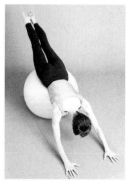

Grasshopper (p. 68)

57. grasshopper

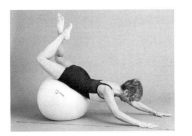

➤ **Stand at the Wall** ➤

Footwork Exercises (p. 81)

58. parallel feet **59. small turnout** **60. high half toe** **61. lower and lift** **62. wide squat**

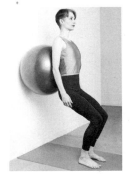 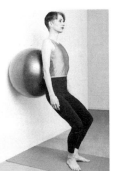 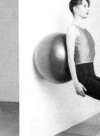 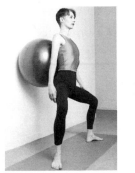 ➤

Leap Frog (p. 83)

63. leap frog

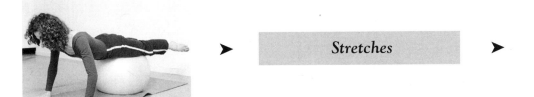

➤ **Stretches** ➤

Shoulder Stretches (p. 117)

64. shoulder shrug   **65. arms overhead**   **66. interlaced fingers**

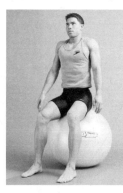 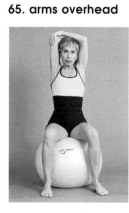 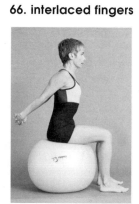

Frog Stretch (p. 110)   Hamstring Stretch (p. 111)   Hip Stretch (p. 112)

67. frog stretch   **68. hamstring stretch**   **69. hip stretch**

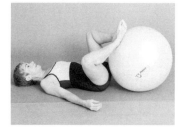 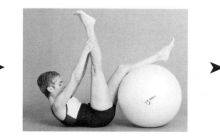 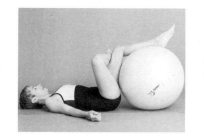

Neck Stretch (p. 113)   The Shell (p. 114)

70. neck stretch   **71. the shell**

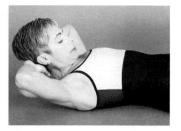 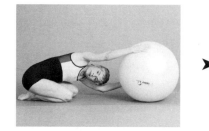

Side Stretches (p. 115)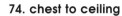

72. side stretch **73. forward stretch** **74. chest to ceiling**

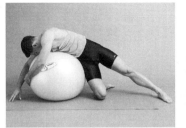

Psoas Stretch (p. 116)

75. psoas stretch

The Arch (p. 118)

76. tabletop with quad stretch **77. the arch**

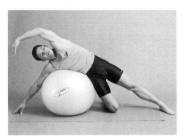

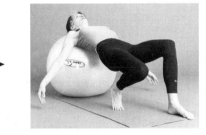

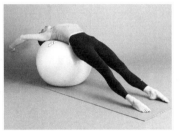

The Squat (p. 120)

78. the squat

De-stressing on the Ball (p. 132)

79. relaxation pose 2 **80. relaxation pose 3**

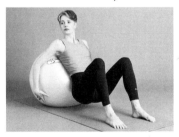

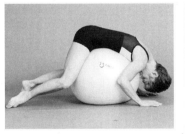

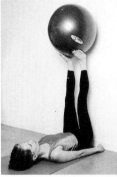

Resources

Books

Calais-Germain, Blandine. *Anatomy of Movement*. Seattle, Wash.: Eastland Press,1993.

Calais-Germain, Blandine, and Andree Lamotte. *Anatomy of Movement Exercises*. Seattle, Wash.: Eastland Press, 1990.

Carrière, Beate. *The Swiss Ball: Theory, Basic Exercises and Clinical Application*. Germany: Springer-Verlag,1998.

Craig, Colleen. *Abs on the Ball*. Rochester, Vt.: Healing Arts Press, 2003.

Hanna, Thomas. *Somatics*. Cambridge, Mass.: Perseus Books, 1988.

Mitchell, Carol. *Yoga on the Ball*. Rochester, Vt.: Healing Arts Press, 2003.

Pilates, Joseph, and William John Miller. *Return to Life through Contrology*. Incline Village, Nev.: Presentation Dynamics Inc.,1998.

Posner-Mayer, Joanne. *Swiss Ball Applications for Orthopedic and Sports Medicine*. Longmont, Colo.: Ball Dynamics International,1995.

Richardson, Jull, and Hides Hodges. *Therapeutic Exercise for Spinal Segmental Stabilization in Low Back Pain*. London: Churchill Livingstone, 1999.

Robinson, Lynne, and Gordon Thomson. *Body Control the Pilates Way*. London: Boxtree, 1997.

Siler, Brooke. *The Pilates Body*. New York: Broadway Books, 2000.

Stark, Steven D. *The Stark Reality of Stretching*. Richmond, B.C., Canada: The Stark Reality Corp.,1997.

Winsor, Mari. *The Pilates Powerhouse*. Cambridge, Mass.: Perseus Books,1999.

Zake, Yamuna, and Stephanie Golden. *Body Rolling: An Approach to Complete Muscle Release*. Rochester, Vt.: Healing Arts Press, 1997.

Videotapes and DVDs

Colleen Craig's On the Ball: An Innovative Ball Video Based on the Work of Joseph Pilates, VHS/color/45 mins. www.pilatesontheball.com

Colleen Craig's Pilates on the Ball™, DVD/color/45 mins. www.pilatesontheball.com

Fitball—Back to Functional Movement by Trish Scott, VHS/color/30 mins.

Fitball—Upper Body Challenge; Fitball—Lower Body Challenge by Cheryl Soleway, VHS/color/45 mins each.

Swiss Ball Applications for Orthopedic and Sports Medicine by Joanne Posner-Mayer, VHS/color/90 mins.

The above videotapes and DVDs can be ordered through Ball Dynamics International or Know Your Body Best; see the following page for contact information.

Ball, Video, and DVD Ordering Information

Ball Dynamics International, Inc.
Makers of Fitball®.

U.S. distributor of exercise balls, *Colleen Craig's On the Ball* videotapes, *Colleen Craig's Pilates on the Ball*™ DVD, and other videotapes and accessories.

800-752-2255
www.fitball.com

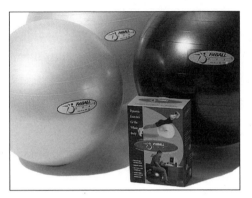

Know Your Body Best
Canadian distributor of exercise balls, *Colleen Craig's On the Ball* videotape, *Colleen Craig's Pilates on the Ball*™ DVD, and therapeutic massage equipment and supplies.

800-881-1681 (in Canada)
www.knowyourbodybest.com

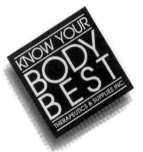

Acknowledgments

I would like to thank my parents, Lorraine and David Craig, and my sister, Jane Welch, for their love and invaluable support. Thanks to my nieces Lyndsey and Lauren, who worked tirelessly with me on the ball, allowing me to learn much from their young, elastic bodies.

Many, many thanks to Laurie Colbert and Dominque Cardona for voluntarily stepping forward to film my video, *On the Ball.* I am grateful to Craig Rose and Marie Jover-Stapinski for appearing with me in the tape and in the book. Thanks also to Claire Letemendia for her editing skills and for cheering me through the writing of the manuscript; Maureen Dwight for her feedback as a physical therapist; Ingrid MacDonald for her sound business advice; David Hou for his wonderful photos and illustrations; and Judd Robbins for sharing his photos of Joseph Pilates. Heartfelt thanks to my editor at Healing Arts Press, Susan Davidson, for superbly editing the final manuscript and for calmly managing the endless details of this project. Thanks to Peri Champine for creating the wonderful cover, to Janet Jesso for doing a fine job with the initial copyediting, and to the rest of the design, production, and marketing team at Healing Arts Press.

I have had many teachers in my ongoing Pilates training, and it is a pleasure to acknowledge them here. I am grateful to Moira Stott for exposing me to and certifying me in Stott Pilates, her contemporary approach to the Pilates Method. I must thank the outstanding senior instructors who were at Stott's at the time of my training, especially Beth Evans, Miriane Braaf, Syl Klotz, Elaine Biagi-Turner, and Connie Di Salvo. In addition, there are those whose movement workshops or videos I have found invaluable: Danielle Belec, Tanya Crowell, Frank Bach, Karen Carlson, Joanne Posner-Mayer, Trish Scott, and Cheryl Soleway. I am indebted to Mari Naumovski for showing me her amazing BodySpheres Ballwork as well as reading the manuscript.

I am most grateful to my sponsors, who have supported my work financially and emotionally from the beginning: Dayna Gutru and all those at Ball Dynamics International and Donna Micallef and Constance Rennett at Know Your Body Best. I want to thank them for supplying the balls and for generously funding the artwork and photographs that appear in this book and on its cover. (Thanks to Constance also for reading the manuscript.)

Over the years there have been key people who believed in me and nurtured me as a writer. They are Robert Harlow, Florence Gibson, Emil Sher, Ingrid MacDonald, Kirsten Strand, Eliza Moore, Rose Scollard, Alexandria Patience, Phillip Kakaza, Edward Shalala, Wayne Morris, Marianne Thamm, Anne Mayne, Vida du Plessis, Helena Scheffler, Christell Stander, and Freddie van Staden. Perhaps most of all I would like to acknowledge Lynne Viola for her emotional support over the years, her expert editorial guidance and career advice, and for taking me with her to wonderful destinations around the world. Also thanks to Monty.

Because I believe that Pilates on the Ball is beneficial to the mind/body as well as the soul, many of my chapter epigraphs are from a book that stresses mind, body, and soul health: *Simple Abundance* by Sarah Ban Breathnach.

Finally, I am most grateful to the students and colleagues who allowed me to change their names and use their stories, or composites of their stories, throughout this book. I am blessed with the most loyal students in the world, and I send many, many thanks to all of you for teaching me new things every day.

Exercise Log

Date	Activity	Comments
half rollup		
Single leg stretch		

Date	Activity	Comments

Date	Activity	Comments

Date	Activity	Comments

Pilates on the Ball™ DVD Directory

Colleen Craig's Pilates on the Ball™ DVD is a carefully designed upper- and lower-body workout consisting of forty-six key exercises selected from the book. There are eight individual workouts of varying lengths, beginning with the Workout Overview or introduction; the DVD is set up so, if pressed for time, you can click on the individual workouts and just do these specific sections.

Some days you might only have time to do the 18-minute Matwork section, a great start to any day. Other days you might want to warm up with the Matwork and add one or two of the shorter sections to your workout. Some days you will want to select the Complete Workout and reap the benefits of the full 45-minute regimen. Take care to always make sure you are fully warmed up before exercising, either by using the Matwork as a warm-up or by doing gentle aerobic movements to heat the body.

It is recommended that you watch the DVD once in its entirety before beginning. This is a basic-level workout with intermediate variations. With the exception of five new exercises that are not shown in the book, each exercise is listed in the facing directory with a corresponding page number so you can refer quickly back to the exercise description in the book. You'll also note in the directory where an exercise is tagged as intermediate—add in these challenging variations only when you are ready. The intermediate exercises are sprinkled throughout the workout, but smaller versions or modifications are usually shown immediately before the more challenging version. Work at your own speed and enjoy your workout.

Workout Overview (2 minutes)

The Matwork (18 minutes)
Breathing (p. 22)
Abdominal Curls (p. 49)
Rollup (p. 52) (Full Rollup is
    intermediate)
Single Leg Circles (p. 54)
The Tree (new exercise)
Obliques (p. 58)
Rolling Like a Ball (p. 55)
Single Leg Stretch (p. 56)
Double Leg Stretch (p. 57)
Lower and Lift (new exercise)
Hip Rolls (p. 93)
Hip Roll Balance (p. 94)
    (intermediate)
Shoulder Bridge Prep (p. 95)
Shoulder Bridge (p. 96)
    (intermediate)
Hip Lift (p. 97) (intermediate; keep
    pelvis down on the mat if
    beginning)
Bend and Stretch (p. 99)
Ball Twist (p. 99) (intermediate)
Ball Balance (p. 101) (intermediate;
    basic level is against the wall,
    p. 134)

Arm Work (4 minutes)
Pulling Arms (new exercise)
Open Shoulder (p. 76)
Hug a Tree (p. 75)
Biceps Curls (p. 76)
Salute (p. 77)
Rowing (p. 78)

Footwork (4 minutes)
Small Turnout (p. 82)
Parallel Feet (p. 82)
High Half Toe (p. 83)
Lower and Lift (p. 84)
Squats (p. 84)
Running (new exercise)

The Postural Exercises
(5 minutes)
Spine Stretch Forward (p. 35)
The Saw (p. 36)
Spine Twist (p. 39)
Mermaid (p. 40)

Extensions (4 minutes)
The Swan (p. 63)
Swan Dive Prep (p. 64)
Swan Dive (p. 65) (intermediate)

Stretches (4 minutes)
The Shell (p. 114)
The Cat (intermediate, new exercise)
Side Stretches (p. 115)

Strength and Coordination
(4 minutes)
Shell on the Ball (p. 66)
Open and Close Legs (p. 67)
Beats (p. 67)
Scissors (intermediate, new exercise)
Push-ups (p. 102)
The Arch (p. 118)

Books of Related Interest

Abs on the Ball
A Pilates Approach to Building Superb Abdominals
by Colleen Craig

Yoga on the Ball
Enhance Your Yoga Practice Using the Exercise Ball
by Carol Mitchell

The Five Tibetans
Five Dynamic Exercises for Health, Energy, and Personal Power
by Christopher S. Kilham

Awakening Kundalini for Health, Energy, and Consciousness
(audiocassette)
by Chris Kilham

Body Rolling
An Experiential Approach to Complete Muscle Release
by Yamuna Zake and Stephanie Golden

The Alexander Technique
How to Use Your Body without Stress
by Wilfred Barlow, M.D.

The Reflexology Manual
An Easy-to-Use Illustrated Guide to the Healing Zones of the Hands and Feet
by Pauline Wills

The Heart of Yoga
Developing a Personal Practice
by T. K. V. Desikachar

Thai Yoga Massage
A Dynamic Therapy for Physical Well-Being and Spiritual Energy
by Kam Thye Chow

INNER TRADITIONS • BEAR & COMPANY
P.O. Box 388
Rochester, VT 05767
1-800-246-8648
www.InnerTraditions.com

Or contact your local bookseller